HOW BAD DO YOU WANT IT?

HOW BAD DO YOU WANT IT?

KAY NYENUH

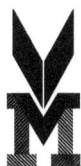

In an Australian context, where many are afflicted by what's called 'tall poppy' syndrome, Kay Nyenuh stands out. Here is a man who is willing to put himself out there as an example for others to follow on the journey towards being better versions of ourselves. We need more people like Kay. *How Bad Do You Want It?* is raw and honest which makes the principles it contains all the more powerful and relatable. The author's background of living in a refugee camp in Ghana gives him unique insights as an observer of Western Culture, which Kay has worked hard to understand. And does the book work? Well I for one have been motivated by it to dust off a few projects I'd given up on – including a set of dumbbells that were sitting around our home unused!

Jai Wright, Founding Pastor of MAKE Church in Mackay and author of Life Plugged In: Connecting with the Source of Peace, Power and Purpose.

How Bad Do You Want It? is a must-read book if you're looking for guidance on your health and fitness journey. Even more importantly, the book provides a how-to for resetting your mindset. What makes *How Bad Do You Want It?* so compelling is the engaging story of Kay's journey from African refugee to Australian small business success story after a chance encounter with a Mackay pensioner. Read it. Use it. Apply it. It's that simple!

Kylie Porter, CEO, Greater Whitsunday Alliance

If you are searching for guidance in getting your life in shape, both physically and mentally, then this book will set you up with the tools to achieve this. Kay explains in simple language how to develop the right mindset for success in all aspects of your life – both personally and professionally; physically and mentally. He delves into his personal experiences and challenges you to understand that anything is possible IF you want it bad enough. There are a lot of personal development books out there but this book is written from his unique perspective in developing the right mindset to live your best life on your terms.

Brendan Keates, Regional Manager – North Queensland, Southern Steel

Jordon and I started training with Kay within two weeks of hearing his first radio ad. We had tried different gyms and personal trainers in town, but something never sat right for us. It was not until we met with Kay for our first consult that we knew what was missing – integrity, honesty, passion, and a genuine heartfelt desire to help people. We ended that consult certain that Kay was the trainer for us and have not looked back. Over the course of the last eight-plus years we have continued to train with Kay and were the first founding members of the Muscle Garden Family. This book *How Bad Do You Want It?* is the distillation of a lifetime to date worth of knowledge and experience, laid out and accessible for anyone who has asked themselves how bad do they truly want something regardless of whether it be health, fitness, or a goal in life. We have seen and witnessed Kay 'talk the talk' and most importantly, walk that talk every day in everything he has done. We are proud and blessed to know Kay as a personal trainer, businessman and owner, and above all as friend and part of our family.

If you have ever asked yourself 'How Bad Do I Want It?' then this is the book for you.

Rachel and Jordon Euler – Founding Muscle Garden Gym and Family Members, Academic Lecturer – CQUniversity School of Nursing, Midwifery and Social Sciences

A story to inspire.

Kay demonstrates by his own personal experience, leading by example, how obstacles are there only for us to work out how to smash them.

This book is not about judgement, instead it is honest and it is acceptance that we are not all equal and do not have the same goals.

It is practical with lots of takeaways, do it yourself guidance and education on how to work out what it is that you want and how to get it.

Nothing is too hard unless you decide it is.

How Bad Do You Want It? is a book about overcoming barriers with implementable steps to do it yourself.

Take the first step to helping yourself by reading it. Highly recommended.

Barb Popp, Founder and Owner, Popp Hand Therapy

I first connected with Kay in 2015 as a PT client. Fast forward five years and I have had the privilege to learn from and train with Kay over that period. I have witnessed Kay develop as a person, work through the many challenges of life and seen his business grow from strength to strength. When he told me he was in the process of writing his first book, I was keen to read it when finished.

Coming from a competitive sporting background, I have read a lot of health and wellbeing and training material. Whether you are someone starting out, part way into your health and wellbeing journey, or a seasoned athlete, I am confident you will enjoy and learn from Kay's book *How Bad Do You Want It?*

In addition to the journey Kay takes you on from his life in Africa, to refugee and starting a new life in Australia. This book is full of great material which you can learn and apply to your health and fitness goals. I found the sections on the right mindset, development and application of goal setting and development of empowering habits, informative and mapped out in a way you can apply, most valuable. I also found the section on nutrition straight forward and easy to understand. The book really is a road map to all you need to be planned, focused, and informed on all aspects of mind, nutrition, and training.

Kay is a person who walks the talk when it comes to living a healthy and active life and leading by example with his family and friends, Muscle Garden family members and the broader community.

If you are ready to change your life or turbo charge your health and wellbeing goals, this book is a must read. How bad do you it, just a little or really bad – go get it!

Scot Alcorn, Territory Manager, Orica

Knowledge is power, and this book delivers on that power.

Unlike other health and fitness books that I have read in the past, *How Bad Do You Want It?* provides the level of detail required to be able to make positive choices about my health and fitness, without any fuss or gimmicks. With the right mindset, the ability to set goals, and the knowledge of the key strategies to action and implement – then, as Kay says 'anything is possible if you want it bad enough'. A great read for anyone wanting to fine tune their health and fitness for the ultimate purpose of leading a more energetic life.

Emily Hayles – Physiotherapist, Business Owner, and Author

First published in 2021 by Kay Nyenuh

A catalogue entry for this book is available from the National Library of Australia.

ISBN: 978-1-922391-73-5

Project management and text design by Michael Hanrahan Publishing
Cover design by Peter Reardon

CONTENTS

FOREWORD

By Mayor Greg Williamson

This is probably the only self-help book you will need to have in your library for the next couple of years. In 256 easy-to-read pages, Kay Nyenuh delivers not just the motivation to get your mind in order, but recipes (peanut butter soup!!) and exercise plans to produce a body capable of letting your mind reach its potential.

There are many books like this on the market, but very few have been underpinned by a personal experience as challenging as Kay's. The credibility of the underlying philosophy in *How Bad Do You Want It?* is his story of growing up in Liberia. Dodging bullets, running for his life as a 10-year-old, 14 years of civil war, living in a refugee camp in Ghana; it makes Kay more than qualified to be able to say that there's two choices in life. 'Wish it would change or change it yourself'.

If you are inclined to 'change it yourself', you will find the blueprint here. Kay deals with creating the right mindset through the messages we give ourselves, and then through nutrition and exercise, giving that mindset energy and vitality to achieve your goals.

The excuses we all use are addressed too. The most common of course is that 'there's not enough time'. There's a section on getting more exercise done in less time. Our relationship with food is great reading and challenges the concept of food being used as a reward or punishment in our society.

Kay's great response to the excuse of 'One day I will start exercising' is that there are seven days in a week and Oneday is not one of them!

Understanding things like Plyometrics and Zercher Squats will have you speaking the language of energy in no time, but the message really is that everything in your life needs to pass through the filter of 'How Bad Do I Want It?' That gives perspective to the true value of the struggle to make yourself a better person.

Greg Williamson
Mayor
Mackay Regional Council

INTRODUCTION

It was not very long ago that I was sitting in a refugee camp in Ghana not knowing where my next meal would come from. If anyone had told me back then that I would move to Australia and in less than three years I would start a successful business and be in the position that I'm in today, I probably would have doubted them. But I strongly believe that anything is possible if you want it badly enough. And if you do get one thing from this book, I hope it would be that. Having this mindset will dramatically change your life.

Have you ever faced a situation or wanted something where you had to sit down and ask yourself: 'How Bad Do I Want It?' For some people this may seem foreign or strange, but for me, this question has helped me get to where I am today. It is a question I apply to everything I have achieved in my life up to this point, including writing this book. 'How Bad Do You Want It?' is not just a question to me anymore, it's a way of life. It is a mindset, a belief that you can achieve anything if you want it bad enough.

Life is not easy, and some would argue that it's not meant to be. When we stop expecting life to be easy, that is when it stops being or ceases to seem so hard. Anything in life – including an abundance of energy and vitality, achieving the best shape of your life both physically and mentally, and being the best role model for your children and loved ones when it comes to their health and wellbeing – is possible if you want it bad enough.

So, my question to you is: 'How Bad Do You Want It?'

WHY YOU SHOULD READ THIS BOOK

If you're an entrepreneur or business owner and you want to get in the best shape of your life, look and feel great about yourself and know that you're setting great examples for your loved ones to follow, then there has never been a better time for you to do so than now.

How Bad Do You Want It? will:

- show you how to develop the right **mindset** to be unstoppable and believe that you can do anything you set your mind to

- show you how to set and achieve your health and fitness **goals**

- provide **nutritional** advice that makes eating healthily easy and not a chore

- show you what to do when it comes to **exercise** and exercise programs that will give you the most energy and best physical appearance in the least amount of time possible

- teach you how to break bad **habits** and form new and beneficial ones that will help you stay on track

- give you an understanding of how to schedule and prioritise your **time** so that you go from being time poor to having an abundance of time for the things that are most important to you.

When applied, the lessons learned from this book will help you do business and family life at your optimum potential.

WHO IS THIS BOOK FOR?

In working closely with over 500 entrepreneurs and business owners and thousands of everyday people, I've discovered that the majority of them, though excellent at what they do, have three major problems:

1. **They lack energy and vitality.** They feel tired, lethargic or drowsy, and cannot get through their working day without having multiple cups of coffee. Not having energy and vitality means that by the time they get home from work, they are exhausted and have no energy left to play with their children or spend quality time with their partners.

2. **They are not happy with their physical appearance.** They look in the mirror and they do not like what they see. But they are too busy working on their careers, putting everyone and everything else first, and they have not stopped to make time for their own health and wellbeing. And because they are not happy with their physical appearance, it affects their confidence and sometimes their performance.

3. **They feel like they are not setting good examples for their children.** They understand that more than anything else, children copy the examples of their parents. Their lack of exercise and poor food choices is having an impact on their children, and this worries them.

This book is for the driven everyday person who is sick of feeling tired, lethargic, or drowsy and who cannot get through their working day without multiple cups of coffee. It is for someone who wants to get in the best mental and physical shape of his or her life. Someone who wants to find ways to have abundant energy and vitality so they can be more alert and productive at work. And to also have more energy to be able to run around with their children and be able to entertain their partner after work.

It is for the everyday person who wants to look in the mirror and be happy with what they see. Someone who is willing and ready to challenge himself or herself to achieve the best shape of their life; because when you look good you feel good. When you are happy with your physical appearance, you exude confidence, which helps you to perform at your best.

This book is for the everyday person who wants to be a positive role model in the lives of their children when it comes to their health and wellbeing. It is for someone who understands that children copy their parents and someone who is willing to challenge themselves to set good examples in terms of what they eat and to take up physical activity that their children or loved ones can be inspired to do.

WHAT THIS BOOK IS GOING TO DO FOR YOU

In this book you will learn about my 'How Bad Do You Want It? Method' – a method that has been so successful with many of my clients over the years that I have decided to share it in this book for your benefit. It is a six-step guide that when applied will help you achieve the best shape of your life both mentally and physically, and will also help you perform at your optimum potential in both your work and family life.

The 'How Bad Do You Want It? Method' described in this book will take you through the six steps of:

1. Lock in the right mindset for success

2. Set goals that will get you what you want

3. Include good nutrition for a healthy and happy life

4. Get lots of exercise to live a life full of energy and vitality

5. Nail your habits so you can live an effective life

6. Get your time back so you can live life on your own terms

We will examine these steps in detail, but let's take a quick look at each of them now.

1. Lock in the right mindset for success

You will learn how to develop a positive 'How Bad Do You Want It?' mindset that will help you achieve any goal you put your mind to. You will also learn how I have managed to achieve the best shape of my life and build a successful fitness business as well as creating for myself the life I now live when not very long ago I was sitting in a refugee camp feeling hopeless and helpless.

2. Set goals that will get you what you want

You will learn the importance of goal setting and how to set and achieve goals that are important to you and your loved ones. Though this step will be centred on health and fitness goals, the principles learned can be applied to all areas of your life. You will learn how to harness the power of knowing that it's not where you are today in your life that matters, but where you want to be and how bad you really want to get there. You will also learn how to plan and execute your fitness goals.

3. Include good nutrition for a healthy and happy life

I have found that the reason why the majority of people struggle to lose weight and keep it off is because they do not enjoy eating healthily or they find it too hard. In this step you will learn tips and tricks that will make eating healthily an enjoyable part of your lifestyle as opposed to it being a chore. You will also have a meal plan to follow as well as some of our beloved family recipes.

4. Get lots of exercise to live a life full of energy and vitality

In this step I will show you how to make exercise fun. You will learn the importance of exercise and how to get more done in less time, as well as receiving some of my go-to exercise programs for you to do both at home and in the gym.

5. Nail your habits so you can live an effective life

You will learn how habits are formed. You will also learn habits that will enable you to take control of your life. I will show you how to break bad habits relating to your health and wellbeing, and how to develop good ones that will help you look and feel great and have an abundance of energy.

6. Get your time back so you can live life on your own terms

Now is always the right time to make a change, and in this step I will help you discover the things that are most important to you so you can go from being time poor to having an abundance of time for those things that matter most. You will be empowered to say 'no' to things that are of lesser value to you because of a bigger 'yes' you have burning inside of you for things that are of higher importance.

WHO AM I?

My name is Kay Nyenuh. I am the Founder and Owner of Muscle Garden Health & Fitness Centre. I am a Personal Trainer and I specialise in helping business owners go from just existing to LIVING their best lives.

I started Muscle Garden in 2012 as a personal training business, working with clients in parks around Mackay. Today we are grateful to be in two fully equipped 24/7 state-of-the-art fitness facilities with an extremely high reputation in town.

I am a husband, father, and a business owner myself, so I understand the demands and importance of being on top of your game. I have been a fitness fanatic for over 20 years, and at the writing of this book I have been in business for a little over eight years. During this time, I have put in over 13,000 hours working one on one with more than 500 entrepreneurs and business owners at my business Muscle Garden, to help them transform not only their bodies but also the way they think and feel.

I have been recognised by my local council as a fitness ambassador, given a TEDx Talk, and I have appeared multiple times on Channel 7, Channel 9, SBS and ABC. I have also featured on national radio stations like Hit FM, Triple M, ABC Radio as well as in newspaper and magazine articles and on websites like BuzzFeed.

Having survived 14 years of civil war and multiple refugee camps to become a renowned health and fitness ambassador today, I have distilled my knowledge and experience into *How Bad Do You Want It?* to inspire and help the everyday person – entrepreneur or not – break through both mental and physical barriers to achieve the best shape of their lives and perform at their optimum potential.

So, let's get started with step 1: Lock in the right mindset for success.

STEP 1

LOCK IN THE RIGHT MINDSET FOR SUCCESS

WHAT *IS* A MINDSET?

'Mindset' has many definitions, but they all point to the same thing. Let's look at some of those definitions:

- the established set of attitudes held by someone

- a person's way of thinking and their opinions

- a fixed mental attitude or disposition that predetermines a person's responses to and interpretations of situations.

Regardless of which definition works best for you, your mindset is simply the way you think, your beliefs and attitudes towards situations in life. What is your belief when it comes to your health and wellbeing? What opinions do you hold? And what are your attitudes as a result of your beliefs and opinions?

DO YOU HAVE A FIXED OR GROWTH MINDSET?

The world-renowned Stanford University Psychologist Dr Carol Dweck, in her book *Mindset: The new psychology of success*, points out that an individual either has what she calls a 'fixed mindset' or a 'growth mindset'. According to Dr Dweck, people with a fixed mindset believe that their abilities, skills, intelligence, and potential are fixed and are unchangeable traits. On the other hand, people with a growth mindset believe that their abilities, skills, intelligence, and potential can be developed over time through dedication and hard work.

Being a Personal Trainer, I've seen clients who are dominant in each of the two mindsets. And I have found the ones who have a fixed mindset struggle with processing slow progress, or even no progress for a period of time. They take it personally as a failure, and unfortunately this can completely take them off track. On the other hand, those with a growth mindset seek to identify areas they can improve on. They look back on their week to see where they could make some changes. They work harder and they push themselves harder to get the results they want.

Let's look more closely at each of these.

A fixed mindset

According to Dr Dweck, people with a fixed mindset are afraid of failure. They see failure as the end of their abilities, and it is hard for them to see beyond that. They have to either be good at something or that is the end of it. They believe their abilities, skills and talents are innate and unchanging. They also believe they can either do something or they cannot.

They do not like to be challenged. They believe their potential is predetermined and they take feedback and criticism personally. And they also like to stick to what they know, and they give up easily.

For example, a person with a fixed mindset would say, 'I am not a runner. I have never been, even from when I was younger, so I am not going to bother.'

A growth mindset

Dr Dweck also points out that people with a growth mindset see failure as an opportunity to grow. They believe they can learn to do anything they want. They embrace challenges because it helps them to grow. They believe hard work, effort and attitude determine their abilities. They use feedback constructively and are inspired by the success of others. They believe that if someone else can achieve a goal, they too can do it. And they like to try new things.

For example, a person with a growth mindset would say, 'I am not a runner, but you know what? No one was born a runner so I am going to give it a try, and with time and effort, I too can be a runner.'

* * *

So, do you have a fixed mindset or a growth mindset? Clearly having a growth mindset is the desirable of the two mindsets here, but if you have a fixed mindset, the good news is you can learn to have a growth mindset. The truth is many people have elements of both mindsets. Dr Dweck found that you could have different mindsets in different areas. For example, you might think your personality is fixed but that your intelligence can be developed, or that your social skills are fixed but your creativity can be developed. The mindset you possess in certain areas will determine and guide your attitude and actions in that area.

According to Dr Dweck, mindsets are just beliefs. They may be powerful beliefs, but they are in your mind. And you can decide to change your mind regardless of how hard it may seem.

THE BELIEFS THAT I LIVE BY

I believe I would not be where I am today if it were not for my mindset. And the beliefs that I live by shape my mindset. Though you will find them explained in various parts of this book, here is a list of some of the beliefs that govern my attitudes and responses to situations in life:

- Everything I do in life must pass through the 'How Bad Do I Want It?' test.

- The future can be better than the present, and I have the ability to make it happen through dedication and unwavering determination.

- Anything is possible if I want it bad enough. Where there is a will, there is always a way.

- You can either sit down and wish for your life to change, or you can get up and change it. If it is going to happen, it is up to me.

- Don't say: 'It can't be done'. Ask: 'How can it be done?' or 'Who can help me do it?'

- The human body is a garden of muscles. I must strive to be a good gardener.

- No obstacle is too big! Every challenge is an opportunity to learn and grow and thrive.

- No plan B's – plan B's distract from plan A's.

- Family is not always blood.

- It's not supposed to tickle. Expecting things to be easy in life is a recipe for failure. I need to brace myself for the difficult and the unexpected.

- Hard work beats talent when talent does not work hard. Talent alone is never enough.

- Nobody was born with a tag around their neck to determine what they will become in life. I can be, do and have anything in life if I want it bad enough.

- No cotton candy. No excuses. If I want 50% of the results, then I should put in 50% effort.

- Don't let people with small minds convince you that your dreams are too big. All dreams do come true when we have the courage to pursue them.

- Golden rule: I must strive to always treat others the same way I would want to be treated.

- God is love. 'For God so loved the world that He gave his only Son, that whoever believes in him shall not perish but have eternal life.' John 3:16.

THE STORIES WE TELL OURSELVES BECOME OUR REALITY

I often hear people say:

- 'I can't do this.'

- 'I can't do that.'

- 'I am not smart enough.'
- 'I am not good enough.'
- 'I am not fit enough.'
- 'I am not strong enough.'
- 'I am not fast enough.'
- 'I don't have time.'
- 'I just can't stop eating.'
- 'That is just the way I am.'
- 'Technology is not my thing.'

And on and on and on it goes ...

We tell ourselves all these stories because they make us feel comfortable. Because they do not challenge us. We lower the bar for ourselves so that others will not expect much from us. We limit ourselves. We tell ourselves these stories long enough that they become our realities. Then we wonder why the needle will not shift in our favour. Until we change our mindsets and the way we see ourselves, as well as the lenses through which we see the world and life in general, we will continue to live in the reality of the stories we tell and believe about ourselves.

When you say, 'I can't do this', your brain shuts down. End of story. It does not think any further. But when you say, 'I can', your brain opens up. It goes to work and begins to look for ways, opportunities, and possibilities to help you achieve whatever it is that you may be after. Understandably, it is easy to say 'I can't' because that requires no effort. Saying 'I can' requires effort, energy, and taking responsibility. It requires us to grow into the person who is capable of achieving that which we want.

One of the greatest traits about being human is that, among other things, we have two powerful abilities in our favour: growth and potential. We start life as an embryo and we grow, we evolve, and we have the enormous potential to adapt to any situation and circumstance in life. But sometimes the self-limiting stories we tell ourselves hold us back. And until that changes, we will not really be able to live life to our fullest potential and on our own terms.

IT'S NOT WHERE YOU ARE IN YOUR LIFE TODAY THAT MATTERS ...

Perhaps one of my most powerful beliefs that I wholeheartedly live by is that it's not where you are in your life today that matters but where you want to be and how bad you really want to get there. This is a saying I have told myself many times through all the difficult circumstances life has thrown at me right from a young age. It is easy to give up when it seems like there is no hope. It is at these junctures that many people doubt themselves. They look at their present situation or condition and say things like: 'I don't think I can do it', 'I'm not good enough', 'What have I done to deserve this?'

Your present situation may cause you to doubt yourself and not believe in your abilities. But let me tell you this: so long as you remain in that mindset, nothing will change. For you to rise above your situation, for you to get to where you want to be, you have to change your way of thinking. You have to believe that, 'Yes, this is where I am today, but this is not the end of my story. I am not there yet.' If you want to be something you have never been before, you have to do something you have never done before. You have to pick yourself up regardless of your current situation and work towards achieving that goal you want because anything is possible if you want it bad enough. But it has to start in your mind even when it seems like there is no way out.

MY STORY

I was born in Liberia – a tiny country on the West Coast of Africa. It's the oldest independent nation on the continent of Africa, and it was founded by the United States of America to resettle freed slaves after slavery was abolished there. Unfortunately, Liberia went through 14 years of civil war and so I experienced war at a very young age. This is part of the reason why I am in Australia today.

At the writing of this book, I have been living in Australia for over 11 years. I became an Australian citizen in 2014. Today I am married to my beautiful wife Jessica with three adorable children Malachi, Rosa and Korrioh, and I run a successful health and fitness business: Muscle Garden.

Prior to moving to Australia in 2009, I lived in Buduburam Refugee Camp in Ghana as a refugee.

A typical 10-year-old child in Australia or the western world would tell you stories of holidays they have been on with their parents, the different theme parks they have visited, and days on the beach. Even my own son Malachi, though he is only five, has already been to New York City three times. I on the other hand did not have that luxury growing up. At a young age I had to run for my life and dodge bullets in order to be alive today.

After the war broke out in Liberia, I found myself in neighbouring Ivory Coast as a refugee. The exact details of how I got there are a little unclear due to my age at the time. From there, when I was a bit older, I moved to Buduburam Refugee Settlement in Ghana where the United Nations had a resettlement program for Liberian refugees. Unfortunately, when I got there, new registrations for the resettlement program had ceased. I found myself in a very hopeless situation.

Life in Africa is quite different to what it is over here in Australia or the western world. My children are young now but when they are a bit older one day my plan is to take them to Africa so they can understand what life is really like over there. For example, most people in Africa do not have washing machines or dishwashers. In fact, some do not even know what washing machines or dishwashers are. I used to wash my clothes and wring them out with my hands. I used to wash dirty dishes in tubs filled with water: one for washing and another for rinsing. And depending on how dirty the dishes were, a third tub for further rinsing. The same process was applied to washing dirty clothes.

I remember the first time I used a dishwasher; I placed the containers face up. When the cycle had completed, the bowls were filled up with water.

Unlike my son Malachi, who gets driven to and picked up from school, most students in Africa walk or run kilometres to and from school every day. Most people in Africa do not know what it feels like to flick a switch and have lights turn on. In Liberia, only a small part of the country has electricity, in and around the capital city. You cannot turn on a tap and get running water because you do not have a tap in the first place. Most people have to travel kilometres to get water to drink, cook, clean and shower.

Those are the situations that I grew up in. That was my life. My difficult upbringing helps me to appreciate more what I now have in Australia. And I would love for my children to be able to see that and understand that despite all of those harsh conditions, life still goes on, and hopefully it can help them to appreciate more the little things we take for granted in Australia and the western world.

Happy to be alive

Life as a refugee was tough. I constantly experienced and was surrounded by so much hopelessness and felt helpless most of the time. I lived in makeshift accommodation, slept on the floor, for the most part I did not have a job, and most nights I went to bed not knowing where my next meal was going to come from. And there were many nights I went to bed without having a meal. Have you ever been so hungry that because you had nothing else to put in your mouth, you licked toothpaste, drank some water and went to bed? I have. That was how bad things were. Nonetheless, I was glad to be alive every day. Many people died during the war in Liberia, including relatives of mine, but I was fortunate enough to have survived and this alone was good enough to keep me going, and I sought ways that I could make the most out of the situation I was in.

But, I was not always like that. I too told myself stories about my situation. I started to accept the reality of the situation I was facing. There was a point where I gave up and could not see a way out. And while I was in that mindset, nothing improved. Things got worse and felt harder and more painful. Until one day I decided to change the way I looked at things. I changed what I accepted to be true and real, and created my own reality. And one of the things I did was that against all odds and even though I was not on any resettlement program and did not know anyone who would help me get out of Africa, I began to tell myself first, and then my friends, that one day I would leave this continent of Africa – and when I do, wherever I go, the ground would shake as a sign that a great man has landed. There seemed no possibility of me ever leaving Africa. But I still believed I would one day. And then a miracle happened.

A miracle

My coming to Australia was purely a miracle and something that I dare not take any credit for. But the point I want to make is that I had turned the corner. I had stopped looking at my current situation and accepting it as the end of my story. My mind was prepared, so when the opportunity came, I was ready. Though surprising, my mind had accepted this reality all along. There are many times in life that opportunities present themselves to us that we are not prepared for, so we let them slip by. We never seize the moment. We never make the effort or take the necessary steps to bring those opportunities into fruition because our mindset is not right.

What stories are you telling yourself today, and how are those stories impacting your growth and development?

The start of my entrepreneurial journey

My 'How Bad Do You Want It?' attitude started way back when I was a kid. I remember when I was just a little boy, I used to go around from house to house selling kerosene to people to light their lanterns at night so they could see through the dark. My mum recently reminded me that she bought my first gallon of kerosene and that when I had enough money, I decided to be my own boss. This was before I was even 10 years old. Today, I have a lantern in my office, a replica of what I used to sell kerosene for, as a reminder of the humble beginning of my entrepreneurial journey. As far as I can remember, this was the start of my entrepreneurship.

I also remember that at one point I had a group of friends whose families were in the palm oil business. After school, I would follow my friends to their shop, which was just under 10 kilometres away from where we lived. Our job was to help empty the barrels of oil into smaller containers for people to buy. We would then sell the oil to customers, and our pay was to collect and keep any remnants of oil in the barrels and drums. It was not much; we were literally scraping the bottom of the barrels. But eventually there was enough that we could sell to have some pocket money for school and to get by.

My next venture was a photography business. I started saving some of that money from the palm oil sale to buy a secondhand camera. It took me a while, but I eventually got there. I then became an unqualified photographer. I would take photos of my fellow students, friends and anyone who wanted their photos taken and develop the films and charge them for the photos. Luckily, the photos did not have to be photoshopped or edited back then. I was not always successful though; sometimes I would mistakenly expose the films to light and the photos would be ruined. And I would have disappointed customers, and I myself would be terribly upset. Where were SD cards back then? The money was not much but it helped me survive.

As I grew up there were many other survival business ventures along the way, one of which is part of the reason why I am in Australia today.

I took courses in information technology, and after I had completed my courses, I started to do work for people teaching them basic IT skills like how to use a computer or browse the internet, using Windows and Microsoft Office, designing documents, installing software and so on. I then got a job working at an internet cafe – which by the way served no coffee, tea or cakes. Basically, they were places you go and pay money to use the internet. There, while browsing the internet and chatting through a platform called PalTalk one night, I met Denise Rougier in a Christian chat room. Denise thought Australia would be a great place for me, and she helped me migrate to Australia. More on this story in step 2.

What my experiences taught me is that regardless of how bad situations are in your life, you have two choices. You can either sit down and wish for your life to change, or you can get up and change it. I learnt resilience and persistence, and there are no substitutes for those. And it made me believe that if I could survive the war, which took millions of lives, and if I could survive life in a refugee camp, then there is not really anything that I cannot do if I want it bad enough. That is my mindset.

It is this belief that saw me take up swimming as an adult. The first time was when I first moved to Australia. Lara, a brilliant migrant support worker at the Mackay Regional Council, shortly after I moved here sought funding for a learn-to-swim program for migrants who had moved to the region. She had realised that unlike in Australia and other western countries, people like me who had migrated from Africa and other third-world countries or places where swimming was not a common practice had not learned how to swim. It was a 10-week program designed to help migrants learn to swim, or at least break their fears around water and learn enough to be safe. At the end of the program I got a certificate – the program had served its purpose. But I still did not feel greatly confident in the water – especially in the deep end of the pool.

The second time I took up swimming was after a client and friend of mine Chris Laval, owner of Ray White Mackay City, bought me a voucher for three private swim lessons. We had just completed a triathlon, and Chris saw that I did not do the swim leg of the triathlon, so he asked, and I told him that I could not swim. He then got me the voucher as a kick-start. After my three lessons I was determined to learn how to swim. So, I sought a swim coach, and luckily for me Steven Rennie – another client of mine – was not only a brilliant swimmer but in his past life had been a swim coach back in Scotland. Steven decided to help me free of charge, even though I offered to pay for his time.

Learning how to swim as an adult was probably one of the hardest things I have done in my life. I found swimming hard because, unlike everything I was used to, I could not just breathe whenever I wanted to. And working hard to stay afloat without adequate supply of oxygen to my muscles due to poor timing made swimming exceedingly difficult. For someone who grew up in Australia and learned how to swim as a kid, this may not be a big deal. But I had tears in my eyes after I swam 50 metres non-stop for the first time, and then went on to swim laps – something that had seemed impossible.

Though Chris got me the voucher because he wanted me to do the swimming leg of my triathlons, for me it was more than that. My wife was pregnant, and we were expecting our first son Malachi. The extra incentive was for me to be able to swim with my son, take him to swimming lessons, play with him in water and be comfortable – all things I have been able to do as a result of stepping outside my comfort zone and pushing through the odds.

Mindsets are just a set of beliefs – powerful beliefs that are formed in your brain – and they have the power to either make you or break you. There is a common saying that if you think you can or if you think you cannot, either way you will be right.

If you are reading this book there is a chance that you are an everyday person, an entrepreneur or business owner, and what I know about entrepreneurs and business owners is that they are generally very driven people, which is why you are reading this book in the first place. You may not have had the background and difficult upbringing that I have had, but you certainly have had to overcome some challenges and difficulties in your life and business to be where you are today. And I strongly believe that if you can do that, if you can run a business and a family, you can definitely achieve your health and fitness goals. You are reading this book because you like change, because you like a challenge, and because you like to improve yourself.

Believe me – anything is truly possible if you want it bad enough.

So, 'How Bad Do You Want It?'

My journey to founding Muscle Garden

Whether it was walking or running kilometres to get to school or playing sports, I have always been active. My favourite sport is basketball and I played up to national level in Ghana.

I did do some weightlifting back when I was in school, but I did not really stick with it. I got back into weightlifting about 2003, and I have not looked back since. At the refugee camp in Ghana, we did not really have a proper gym or equipment. For example, the gym I went to, if you can call it that, was a room in an unfinished building. There was no roof over our heads. We made barbells from steel bars and cement. We did not even know what the weights weighed most of the time, but we just lifted them. We had some steel plates. We made our own benches from timber for doing bench press – sounds dangerous, thinking about it now. We did not have a squat rack or any of the fancy equipment I have in my gyms today.

Your muscles usually do not care how fancy the equipment is, they just need to be worked. And neither did we care – we just lifted. We did bench presses, bicep curls, shoulder presses, pullovers and more. There were not a lot of exercises we could do. But we did what we could regardless. We made the most of what we had at the time. It was a way of passing time and doing some exercise.

The thing that really attracted me to lifting weights was the fact that it worked. Say, for example, when you do bicep curls, your biceps immediately start to swell up – what we call 'hypertrophy', an increase in size of muscle cells due to the blood flow to the area. Even though the results are not instant, you get the sense that what you are doing is working.

I loved doing weights, and before I migrated to Australia, one of the first questions I asked Denise was if there was a gym in the area. I was overly excited when she said yes, and that it was just around the corner from the house. That gym was Souths Gym, which now unfortunately is closed to the public. That gym became my second home – a place where I met some lifelong friends who made settling into a new town and country a little easier.

One of those friends was Ben Courtice. Ben was my training partner at Souths. I still remember when he would hold my legs to spot me with my chin-ups. He introduced me to his circle of friends like Andrew Kidcaff, Adam Robb, Jesse Cheyne, Blair Hill, Anthony Watt and more who welcomed me with open arms.

When I first moved here, I went to the gym a lot, both mornings and evenings. I did not really have a problem spending two hours in the gym working out in the morning and going back in the evening for another two hours. I did that because, firstly, I was amazed to see what a gym really looked like and the variety of equipment I now had at my disposal and the plethora of exercises I could now include in my training regimen. Secondly, my jobs at the time were all casual jobs so I had plenty of time on my hands to be a 'gym junkie', as some later referred to me as.

'Why don't you become a personal trainer?'

It was not long before friends and people that I met at the gym started saying to me, 'Why don't you become a personal trainer?' I used to hear that all the time. Some would even go as far as saying, 'You would be very good at it'. But I never really gave it a second thought because I had other plans for what I wanted to be. Most kids from Africa, when given the opportunity, want to be a doctor, a teacher, a lawyer and the like. I wanted to be a lawyer. My dad was a former magistrate court judge before the war; so, I wanted to sort of follow in his footsteps. In fact, at the time I was studying my diploma of justice administration to make it easier for me to get into a law degree here in Australia. But the idea that if I was a bad lawyer,

I could help make an innocent person go to jail, and on the other hand if I was a good lawyer, I could help make a guilty person walk free, made me feel uncomfortable.

The turning point for me was in 2010 when I was walking through Mount Pleasant Shopping Centre, one of two major shopping centres in Mackay. I saw a man walking through the shopping centre. At first, I thought he was wearing a waist bag, so I had to do a double take, and on the second occasion I realised that he was not actually wearing a waist bag and that in fact it was his belly hanging outside of his shirt. Sadly, he was the biggest person I had ever seen in my life.

I immediately felt sad for this man. I said to myself if I could train for this guy so that he could lose weight I would, but unfortunately you cannot train for other people – they have to do it for themselves. So, then I thought if I was to be of any help to this guy – or any other person for that matter – then I had to become a personal trainer.

So I made the decision to follow my passion, because I truly wanted to help people achieve their health and fitness goals and also because it was something I could see myself doing every day with a smile on my face. Growing up in a refugee camp and being surrounded by so much helplessness, I had developed a genuine passion for helping people, and becoming a personal trainer was a way for me to combine my passion for helping people with my love for health and fitness.

Even though I had a lot of people saying to me, 'Why don't you become a personal trainer?', that was not the reason I did so. But at the same time, I did not completely ignore what they were saying. In 2016, I remember speaking to some 200 Year 12 school leavers at St Patrick's College, and I told them this story and reminded them that there will be times in their lives when people will see certain qualities or potentials in them and point those out. My advice to them was to not just jump into doing something because someone told them to. I encouraged them to find their own conviction as to why they want to do it. To sit down and ask themselves, 'How Bad Do I Want It?', because when things get tough – and trust me, they will – that is what is going to keep them going.

I had to be truly clear for myself that personal training was what I wanted to do. I asked myself, 'How Bad Do I Want It?' I realised that I wanted it badly enough that I was willing to dedicate the rest of my life to it.

The launch

On 16 April 2012 while sitting at the Brisbane Domestic Terminal feeling all nervous and excited at the same time, I launched Muscle Garden Personal Training online. I did not want to see the initial reaction, so I did it just before I hopped on the plane, so that by the time I landed in Mackay and got off the plane the news would have already spread across my social media networks.

Starting Muscle Garden was a big decision. Anyone who has started a business would understand. As Reid Hoffman, Co-Founder of LinkedIn, brilliantly put it: 'An entrepreneur is someone who jumps off a cliff and builds a plane on the way down.'

The thing is, it doesn't always work. You do not always get to finish building that plane and instead you hit the ground hard. This gave me some questions that I had to answer for myself, and the two most important ones were:

- **You can train yourself to achieve results, there is no doubt about that, but are you going to be able to translate this to others for them to achieve their own goals?** For such a hard question my answer, as simple as it could be, was the old adage, *I would never know if I did not try*. There was a part of me that believed I could do it and there was also a part of me that doubted. There was only one way to find out.

  'I learned that courage was not the absence of fear, but the triumph over it. The brave man is not he who does not feel afraid, but he who conquers that fear.' – Nelson Mandela

- **What if this Muscle Garden thing does not work out?**
  How are you going to manage? Again, this was another big
  question considering the risk of failure, and the shame and
  humiliation that come with failure and the feeling of rejection.
  How was I going to survive? I had spent my savings on building
  a website and paying for advertising, and I only had enough
  money to live for two weeks. And yet again my answer was
  remarkably simple but so profound, and it could not have been
  any clearer in my mind. My answer was, if it did not work out at
  the start, I had the rest of my life to make it work. For me there
  was no Plan B. Not everyone will agree with this, but I believe
  Plan B's distract from Plan A's. There was no turning back for
  me. I had to give it my absolute best. Everything and whatever
  it took to make it work. Having nothing to fall back on gave me
  every bit of motivation and the desire I needed to be successful.

I could not even begin to tell you all about the incredible results my
clients have achieved since starting Muscle Garden in 2012, but I will
share some of the case studies to help demonstrate the steps in this
book. Today I make a living doing what I love, and it's truly a beautiful thing and a blessing when a passion and a career come together.

It was a bumpy road

But it was not always as it is today.

When I started Muscle Garden Personal Training, I did not have
a gym to work from. I approached gyms in town to see if they would
let me train my clients out of their facilities for a fee, but even though
I was going to pay them, even though I was bringing them business,
they all refused. One of the owners even said to me, 'Why don't
you come and work for me?' The fact is if I wanted to work for anyone, I would not have bothered starting a business in the first place.
I started Muscle Garden because I had a set of values, principles,
and ways of doing things that I did not believe I could carry out had
I worked for someone else. And for me this was my first test.

The refusal of the gym owners was not personal. Knowing what I know now and how I run my business, I too would politely say no to a young aspiring personal trainer who wanted to run her business out of my gym, due to the conflict of interest.

I used their refusal to fuel a fire inside of me to start my own gym. But before I started my own gym, I worked out of a friend's gym. A buddy of mine, Kris Hayho, had just opened Star Bodies. We both started our businesses around the same time, and we realised that we could benefit from each other. So, we struck a deal; my clients would become members of his gym and I would train them at his facility.

But I still had a burning desire to open my own gym. I saw a gap in the market, and I did not like how most gyms were run. I did not like how people were treated just like another number, how no one cared if you showed up or not. I did not like how everyday people felt intimidated to go to the gym, how they felt out of place. I did not like that there was not a support network. I did not want my personal training clients walking into those environments after they had finished their personal training packages with me. So, I decided to open a gym for the everyday person, the everyday mums and dads. A gym that is welcoming – where members are greeted by their names when they walk in. A gym that is family-oriented – where members feel part of a support network bigger than just a gym. And one that is free of any form of intimidation – where members feel comfortable to train.

In 2013, sixteen months after I started Muscle Garden Personal Training, I opened my first gym: Muscle Garden Health & Fitness Centre on Wood Street in Mackay. The total floor space was about 95 square metres. It was small! But we made it work. And amazingly enough, the majority of those members from back then are still our members today.

In November 2014, we faced a challenge. We were given a month's notice to vacate the premises. I had a month-to-month agreement with my previous landlord who had gone bankrupt, and the real estate agent told me the new owner did not want a gym in his building – something I later found out to be untrue.

So, we had to move. It was an incredibly stressful time. My wife was pregnant with our first child. We had just gotten married two months earlier, and we had our honeymoon to New York planned for December to visit my mum and aunty as well as other family members. We had to cancel our honeymoon to find a new location for the gym. As stressful as it was at the time and without knowing where we were going, I believed we were going to be in a bigger and better place. So, I sent out an email to my clients and gym members telling them that we were moving to a bigger and better place. As things worked out, almost 16 months after I opened Muscle Garden Health & Fitness Centre, we moved into a bigger space at 157 Victoria Street.

Anything is possible if you want it bad enough.

10 COMMON MISTAKES AND HOW TO OVERCOME THEM

Below are 10 thinking mistakes people make when it comes to their health and wellbeing, the actions they take as a result of such thinking, and why this is a problem. And also the mindsets they should adopt to achieve a lasting change.

Thinking mistake 1: I do not have time to exercise

Action: They do not make time to exercise.

Problem: Not making time for exercise is a problem because research shows that inactivity contributes to 6% of all deaths globally. It is a problem because not making time for exercise is essentially making time for illnesses. Lack of exercise contributes to a cluster of health-related problems, including but not limited to osteoporosis, being overweight or obese, poor sleeping patterns, depression and anxiety, heart attacks, type 2 diabetes, low self-esteem, and lack of energy and vitality.

Mindset to achieve lasting change: Make time for exercise. Prioritise your health. You cannot afford the consequences of neglecting your health.

Take Stephen for example: Stephen was a 55-year-old co-owner of a mine site service business. Before he joined Muscle Garden his thinking was: I work 12- to 15-hour days and I do not have time to exercise. As a result of this thinking, Stephen avoided exercise or did not make time to exercise. This was a problem because, as mentioned above, research shows that inactivity contributes to 6% of all deaths globally and a cluster of other health problems.

Stephen's weight got up to 140-plus kilograms, and one day he found himself on a hospital bed. His doctor warned him that he needed to lose weight if he wanted to be around longer. Stephen then tried a few different fitness centres and personal trainers before coming to Muscle Garden.

During my consultation with Stephen I explained to him that I had one hour in a day to work with him. He had 23 hours on his own. Whatever he did within those 23 hours would make the one hour spent with me worthwhile. I also explained to him that I reserved the right to say no to clients if I saw that they were wasting their money and my time. It was something that stuck with Stephen. It was important for me to explain these things to Stephen because I really wanted him to buy into why he was starting this journey.

I then asked him when he would like to start. He said, 'Today if you have time'. Two hours later I conducted Stephen's fitness assessment. We spent more time recovering than we did on the actual assessment. Stephen knew he was in a bad shape and he was not going to stop until he had achieved his goals.

Stephen, who once thought he did not have time for exercise, found a way and made time for exercise. He now wanted it badly enough. Some mornings I would get to work at 4:45am for Stephen's 5am session and he would already be there waiting for me after driving in from over 30 kilometres away.

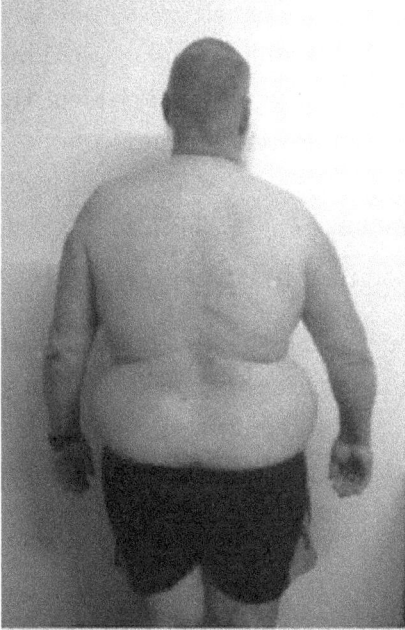

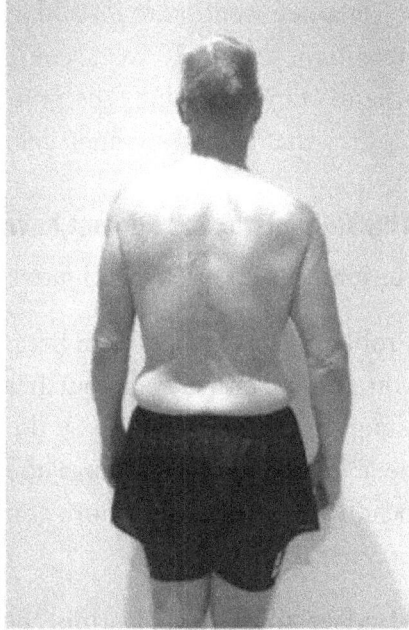

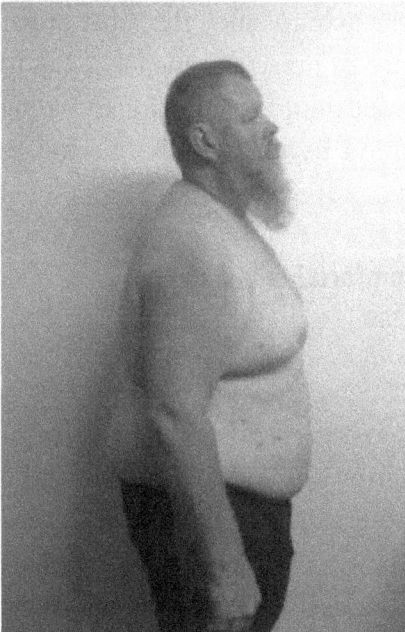

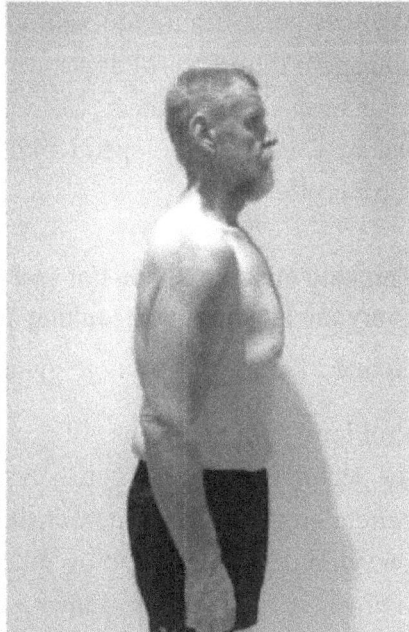

Before and after photos of Stephen

Stephen went on to lose 56 kilos of body fat. He ran for the first time in more than 20 years, competed in triathlons, and inspired his wife to start exercising. His productivity at work was sky high. He told me that he had so much energy that he found it hard to stop.

Thinking mistake 2: I do not have money

Action: They do not spend money on their health and wellbeing.

Problem: This is a problem because usually what this means is that you are not prioritising your health. You can have all of the finest things in the world but if you do not have good health, you will not be able to enjoy those things abundantly or enjoy them at all. Your health should be your priority and it should not come at the mercy of other things.

Mindset to achieve lasting change: Your health is your wealth. Without good health you will not be able to enjoy that boat or car you spent thousands of dollars to buy. Be proactive when it comes to your health and wellness. Do not wait until something goes wrong before you decide to spend money on health. Usually this way is most costly.

Thinking mistake 3: I do not feel comfortable in a gym; everyone is going to be looking at me

Action: They avoid going to gyms.

Problem: Avoiding gyms is a problem because it creates a barrier for the person feeling this way to access an environment where they could benefit from using a range of different exercise equipment. It also prevents them from tapping into the experience of knowledgeable staff who could help them improve their self-esteem and confidence. And hiding as a result of thinking 'everyone is going to be looking at me' is a problem because in most cases that's not true. People often go the gym for their own personal reasons.

Mindset to achieve lasting change: Do not avoid gyms; find one that has a friendly, supportive, and welcoming environment that is free of intimidation. One that cares more about helping you achieve your health and fitness goals than they care about profit making.

Thinking mistake 4: I will wait until I get fit first before I see a personal trainer or join a gym or do a boot camp

Action: They try to do it on their own with little or no success.

Problem: Trying to do it on their own is a problem because most times, even though it may seem like the cheaper option at first, it can be very costly:

- *It costs time:* the person is trying to learn through their own mistakes instead of learning from those who are already experts in the field and have made and learned from many mistakes themselves. It sometimes takes them longer to get to their goals, if they get there at all.

- *It costs money:* the person is buying home gym equipment and accessories that they will not use long term due to lack of accountability and loss of motivation. The equipment ends up collecting dust and taking up space.

- *It costs functionality:* the person is injuring himself or herself and not able to function properly, which can also lead to feelings of depression and anxiety.

Mindset to achieve lasting change: Do not wait until you get fit first before you see a personal trainer or join a gym or a boot camp. Just start. You do not have to be good to start but you have to start if you want to be good. And secondly, you do not have enough years in your life to learn from your own mistakes. Get help. You see professionals for almost everything else in your life. Why not with your body?

Thinking mistake 5: When I lose weight then I will be happy or love myself

Action: They have an attitude of self-loathing.

Problem: This is a problem because true happiness or self-love comes from within not from without. Yes, losing some weight will boost your self-esteem and confidence, but if your happiness or self-love are tied to that then you will never truly be happy or love yourself and this can lead to other problems. In addition, self-loathing can cause unnecessary worrying and anxiety, which can sabotage one's actions and motivation.

Mindset to achieve lasting change: Self-love first, then the rest will follow. If you do not start by loving yourself first, even when you achieve that weight loss you still will not be happy with yourself. Start from the inside out. Everything that we need is already within us.

Thinking mistake 6: I eat pretty healthily

Action: They go about their day eating foods that they perceive to be healthy because of smart marketing of products labelled organic, 99% fat free and no added sugar or preservatives.

Problem: Misleading packaging and misinformation is causing people to think they are making healthy food choices, however this may not be the case. And as a result, this affects their weight, mood, energy levels, sleep and many other things. It's also a problem because for those with children, this misinformed eating can be passed down to children, creating a vicious cycle. (For more on this, see step 3, Include good nutrition for a healthy and happy life.)

Mindset to achieve lasting change: Make informed decisions. See a nutritionist or dietician. Get help.

Thinking mistake 7: All things in moderation

Action: They consume unhealthy food and drinks on occasion.

Problem: Eating and drinking junk food with the mindset that a little bit here and there will not hurt you is a dangerous problem because what the person with this mindset doesn't see is that big things really do come in small packages. All the small amounts of bad food and drink here and there add up, and over time they contribute to a bigger problem that needs time to be solved. What I have found with this problem is that people are not honest with themselves. Surely if you are truly having just a little bit of junk food or drink once in a blue moon, that is not enough to hurt you? But I have seen people with this thinking consume junk food or drink on a daily and weekly basis.

Mindset to achieve lasting change: Willpower is key here. The brain is a muscle – the more you exercise it the stronger it will get. But like every muscle, the more you use it, the more it fatigues. In this case avoiding the temptation is sometimes better than relying on willpower alone. Out of sight, out of mind works magic. This will not happen overnight, and it is going to take practice, determination and perseverance. But you can do it.

Thinking mistake 8: I have tried everything; nothing works

Action: They give up.

Problem: Giving up is a problem because they have tried everything but one. Sticking it out. Giving it heart and effort when the going gets tough. If we think about how many years we have spent taking our body for granted, we will understand that results are not going to happen overnight. Perseverance and consistency are key.

Mindset to achieve lasting change: Never give up. Even if you do not see the results you are seeking for a long time, keep going.

You are more likely to achieve your results when you keep going versus when you stop. Winners never quit and quitters never win.

Thinking mistake 9: I can exercise whenever I choose and still get results

Action: They exercise sporadically without any routine or schedule.

Problem: This is a problem because someone with this mindset does not have the right habits or a system in place to help them achieve their goals. It is also part of the reason why a lot of people sign up for gym memberships but don't go as much as they should. I hear stories of how people signed up for a 12-month contract and only attended the gym once or twice. I have also seen members of my gym who – despite all our efforts contacting them and trying to get them back into the gym – have not been for over 12 months. Exercising whenever you choose will not help you get the results you desire.

Mindset to achieve lasting change: Have a system and a routine. Plan your week in advance. Pick the days and times that you will exercise and schedule them in and set reminders. And stick to it. Some days will not always go according to plan but at least you will *have* a plan. After a while this becomes a habit. It becomes automatic. For example, if you work out at 6am every Monday, Wednesday and Friday, after a while you would know what this time is for, and if you don't work out then, you would feel something is missing.

Thinking mistake 10: My goal is to lose weight, get fit or get stronger

Action: They sign up for a gym membership or take up some form of training.

Problem: This is a problem because saying I want to lose weight, I want to get fit or I want to get stronger is not a goal. It is a wish, and wishes do not get results.

Mindset to achieve lasting change: Set a goal with specific details. Identify what you want and why you want it. And then how you are going to achieve it. What are the possible challenges you are going to face? What identity are you going to adopt? What kind of person is capable of achieving the goal you want? And what are you going to do every day to make sure you achieve that goal?

I want to lose weight – how much weight and by when?

I want to get fit – what would this mean for you? What is 'fit'? be clear about what you want. And when you want it.

I want to get strong – how strong? What do you want to be able to do that will make you know that you are strong? And by when? (For more on how to set goals that will get you what you want, see step 2.)

Your mind is the most powerful tool you have at your disposal. You can either use it to your advantage or disadvantage.

SO, HOW BAD DO YOU WANT IT?

'How Bad Do You Want It?' is a mindset. It falls on the side of a growth mindset. People with this mindset believe anything is possible if they want it bad enough. They realise that if they want something bad enough, they will do whatever it takes to get there. They will make sacrifices, avoid making excuses and endure whatever challenges may lie before them to get to their goal. It is a way of life. It is a belief I live by and one that has helped me to get to where I am today.

I have also seen how by adopting this mindset many of my clients have managed to achieve huge goals that at first seemed impossible. Anyone with this mindset can recreate his or her life for the better.

When your mindset is right, everything flows. People with the 'How Bad Do You Want It?' mindset – who believe anything they want in life is possible if they want it bad enough and dedicate themselves to working hard, applying effort, heart and determination – are unstoppable. They are unshakable. They know what they want, and they go out there and get it regardless of circumstances, or what anyone thinks. Even when the going gets tough, they find a way to push through; to persist until something happens; to grind it out until they achieve their goal.

'How Bad Do I Want It?' is a question that most people would not be accustomed to asking themselves before embarking on a journey, taking a course, or doing something new. It is a question I ask myself almost on a daily basis. Basically, everything I have achieved is as a result of first getting very clear on how bad I really wanted it and tying it to the unwavering belief that I can do anything if I want it bad enough. I have developed what I call the 'How Bad Do I Want It?' Test, which has helped me to get crystal clear on everything I've achieved. Here's the test that I use:

THE 'HOW BAD DO I WANT IT?' TEST

1. WHAT DO I WANT?

2. WHY DO I WANT THIS?

3. WHAT CATEGORY DOES IT FALL UNDER – PERSONAL DEVELOPMENT, FAMILY, BUSINESS, OR COMMUNITY?

4. HOW IS IT GOING TO CHANGE MY LIFE OR THE LIVES OF THOSE INVOLVED?

5. WHAT IS THE UPSIDE?

6. WHAT IS THE DOWNSIDE?

7. CAN I LIVE WITH THE DOWNSIDE?

8. HOW MUCH OF MY LIFE WILL I NEED TO GIVE AWAY TO ACHIEVE THIS AND WILL IT BE WORTH IT?

Let's look at just a few examples of the things I've used this test on:

- the decision to become a personal trainer
- the decision to leave the mines and start a business
- the decision to open up a gym
- the decision to learn how to swim as an adult
- the decision to have a family
- the decision to expand my gym
- the decision to write a book.

Most people do not achieve their goals in life because they lack the self-belief and self-confidence that they can do it. Self-belief and self-confidence are the keys to achieving any goal in life. Achieving something worthwhile is not easy. There will be failures along the way. As Winston Churchill once said: 'Success consists of going from failure to failure without loss of enthusiasm.' Having the self-belief that you can do it is imperative for your success. It is this belief that will help you to push through when things get hard.

Many people doubt themselves before they even begin. Never doubt yourself; never think you are not good enough and that you cannot or are not able to achieve your goal. Being human means inevitably those thoughts will cross your mind. We all have imposter syndrome at different times. But you have to rise above it. You cannot let those thoughts hold you back. Napoleon Hill once said: 'Whatever the mind of a man can conceive and believe, it can achieve.' I like to add that while conceiving and believing are essential, action is required for achievement to happen. You must believe that you can and act accordingly.

By adopting the 'How Bad Do You Want It?' mindset, you will be able to figure out what your goal means to you before you start, and the end result – your desired outcome – will become your driving force, your purpose, your why. And it is this drive that will help you become unstoppable regardless of the challenges along the way. It will help you develop resilience and persistence and enable you to persevere until you achieve your goal. Having clarity on your desired result will give you the confidence you need to achieve any goal, including your work or business goals, your personal goals, and your health and fitness goals. You will discover the abundance of energy and vitality to be more productive at work and at home, a physical appearance or body that you are happy with, and a healthy lifestyle that will make you a positive role model for your children and loved ones.

ANYTHING IS POSSIBLE IF YOU WANT IT BAD ENOUGH

Anything is possible if you want it bad enough, and I mean *absolutely anything*. If you can dream it, you can achieve it. This is also another mindset that is imperative to any form of success. For you to achieve anything in life, you have to first believe you can achieve it and then work towards it. As Theodore Roosevelt once put it: 'Believe you can, and you're halfway there.' If you do *not* believe it in the first place, your effort will be lacklustre, and you may never achieve what it is that you want. Most people doubt themselves to start with, and that is the recipe for failure.

You can achieve anything you put your mind to. You do not even have to be what society considers being smart, intelligent, or even have a university degree for that matter. If you believe you can do it, you will find ways, means, people, resources and skills to help you achieve your goal.

The problem is most people just want to be successful. Most people just want to lose weight. Most people just want to be fit and healthy. Most people just want to have abundance of energy and vitality so that they can be more productive at work and be able to run around with their children at home. Most people just want to get in the best shape of their life, to achieve the body they can look at in the mirror and be happy with. Most people just want to be a positive role model and set good, healthy lifestyle examples for their children and loved ones to follow. But the problem is they do not want it bad enough. They do not want it as bad as they want to drink alcohol and eat junk food. They do not want it as bad as they want to watch TV and play video games. They do not want it as bad as they want to spend time on social media. They just want it.

But all that can change. Because it is in your mind, and you can decide to change your mind anytime.

The thing about wanting something bad enough is that the outcome usually outweighs the sacrifices that you have to make. But first you have to get noticeably clear on *why* you want what you want. You have to ask yourself: How Bad Do I Really Want It? Because if you want it bad enough, you will make the sacrifices necessary to achieve your goal and you will do whatever it takes to get there.

STEP 2

SET GOALS THAT WILL GET YOU WHAT YOU WANT

CLARIFY YOUR GOALS TO ACHIEVE WHAT YOU REALLY WANT IN LIFE

After many years of research into how our brains work, scientists were able to discover that for our brains to figure out how to get what we want, we must first decide what it is that we want. Once we lock in our desires through goal setting, whatever goal we give to our sub-conscious mind, the brain will actively start looking for information, resources, opportunities and ways to help us achieve what we want.

What is a goal? Due to the nature of my work (personal trainer, gym owner), I get to ask people almost every day what their goals are for joining the gym, taking up personal training, or doing both. And what I have found is that the majority of people, sometimes through no fault of their own, do not understand what a goal is. And as a result of that, the common answers I hear are:

1. 'I want to lose weight.'

2. 'I want to get fit.'

3. 'I want to tone up.'

4. 'I want to get stronger.'

Now, when you do not understand goal setting you might think those are perfectly fine goals. I mean, they seem totally logical, right? But I want you to pause for a minute and read those again and try to figure out what is missing.

A goal is defined as an **idea** of the **future** that a person or an organisation **envisions**, **plans**, and **commits** to achieve or reach within a **finite timeframe** by setting **deadlines**. Can you start to see what is missing from our examples above?

Based on the definition, there are some key words to consider here. First, it is just an *idea* to start with. It is something that you *envision* – something that you imagine or visualise as a future pos-sibility. And the stronger your emotions are towards that image in your mind, the more likely you are to bring that idea into reality. Thoughts actioned become things and reality.

Secondly, just having the idea in your mind is not enough. You must make *plans* towards achieving that goal. A detailed outline of how you are going to achieve your goal makes working on your goal easier. And by making progress on your plan, you build confidence that you can achieve your goal.

Thirdly, you must *commit* to that goal. Without commitment no goal will be achieved.

And lastly, you must set *deadlines*. A goal without a deadline is just a wish or a good idea. A deadline enables you to focus and work towards achieving your goal within a set timeframe – the beginning and the end. Remember, pressure makes diamonds. But I must also say this, while setting deadlines is especially important, if you do not achieve your goal by a set deadline, it does not mean that you abandon your goal. Do not change the goal, change the timeline or move the deadline until you have achieved that goal, unless it is no longer important to you.

By setting deadlines, you will become good at gauging how long it will take you to achieve a goal you set for yourself in the future.

The issue with 'I want to lose weight, get fit, tone up or get strong' is that though they sound very reasonable, they are not goals. They are what I call good ideas, dreams or wishes.

I will dive a little deeper into this later, but for now let's first understand why it is important to set goals.

WHY IS IT IMPORTANT TO SET GOALS?

It is particularly important for us to set goals because through goal setting you can create for yourself the life you want. The body that you want; the career that you want; the financial status that you want; the life/work balance that you want. I say life/work balance because I do not believe we were put on this earth to prioritise working over living. By setting goals, you will also be able to get the relationship that you want, the personal development, and so much more.

Setting goals gives you a sense of purpose and meaning. And having purpose and meaning in life brings happiness. Achieving goals also helps to boost your self-confidence in your ability to achieve things that are important to you.

WHY DO MANY PEOPLE *NOT* SET GOALS?

So! If goal setting is so important, why is it that many people do not set goals? There are several answers to this question, but I believe these four reasons capture the essence of why people do not set goals:

1. **They think goal setting is not important.** If like me you grew up in an environment where setting goals was not part of your upbringing, you would not consider it. Or you may think it is unnecessary. But the good news is, goal setting can be learned. I learned it and it has made a world of difference to my life.

2. **They do not know how to set goals.** The majority of people genuinely do not know how to set goals. And I used to be one of them. So, when I hear potential clients say, 'I want to lose weight' as their goal, I understand where they are coming from and so I help guide them in the direction of setting and achieving their goals. I help turn their good ideas, dreams and wishes into goals that can be achieved.

3. **They fear failure.** Failure is something we all fear. The fear of failure can be crippling. Failure itself brings upon us both emotional and financial heartaches which can be very painful at times. It is this fear that can limit us in our ability to set big goals, so we often tend to play it safe. We set the bar low. We wallow within our comfort zones. We set Plan B's so that if our Plan A's do not work, we have something to fall back on – which by the way is a sure way to not achieve Plan A. More on this later. What helps me overcome my fears is believing

that courage is not the absence of fear but understanding that something is more important and acting towards that thing is greater than the fear. You never fail, you only learn – if you pay attention. If failure is not an option, then neither is success.

4. **They fear rejection.** We are social beings, and whether we agree with it or not, we value the opinions of others, what they think of us, and we sometimes crave their validation. We fear that if we set a goal and do not achieve it, others will criticise or ridicule us. If you have this concern, my advice is that you first keep your goals to yourself. And as you get more confident in achieving your goals then you can start telling people.

HOW TO SET AND ACHIEVE YOUR GOALS

There are two most important reasons why people never achieve their goals in life. Knowing these two reasons will make a huge difference to you setting and achieving meaningful goals:

1. **They do not know WHAT they want.** You can never achieve something that you do not know. You cannot hit a target that you cannot see.

2. **They do not know WHY they want it.** If you do not have a WHY your chances for success are extremely limited.

In goal setting, it is especially important to first get crystal clear on these two things. Identify:

* WHAT is it that you want? – Your Desire.
* WHY do you want it? – Your Why, Purpose or Drive.

Knowing your WHAT and WHY will help you determine your HOW – how am I going to achieve this goal? Then your WHEN – when do I want or need to achieve this goal by?

And then before you even start working on your goal, you ask yourself what I call the second HOW – How Bad Do I Want It?

Having just a desire is not enough. It must be a burning desire and the size of the fire under your desire must be to the same magnitude as a bush fire.

To determine your WHY, it helps to first ask yourself: how is this going to change my life or the lives of others? What impact or difference will it make if I achieve this goal? See the 'How Bad Do I Want It?' test on page 38.

SMART GOALS

For any goal to be within your grasp or achievable, it must be what is referred to as a SMART goal:

SPECIFIC: Your goal must be truly clear, concise, and well defined.

MEASURABLE: It must be a specific amount by a specific time.

ATTAINABLE: It must be achievable within the constraints of time, money, environment as well as your skills and abilities. It is also good to set goals that will stretch you – breakthrough goals. Do not be afraid to challenge yourself and set goals that will stretch you right outside of your comfort zone.

REALISTIC: Keep your goals in line with your purpose. There is no point setting a goal about something that you are not interested in. If your emotions about that goal are not strong, there is a good chance you will not achieve it. A goal must be aligned with your values, beliefs and principles.

TIME-BOUND: Set deadlines and sub-deadlines. A goal without a deadline is just a wish.

'Set a goal so big that in the process of achieving that goal, you become someone worth becoming.' – Jim Rohn

GOALS VERSUS WISHES

Wish: *I want to lose weight.* I want to lose weight is just a wish or a good idea because it does not meet all the criteria of a goal. As mentioned above, a goal must be specific, measurable, attainable, realistic and time-bound. Can you see what is missing in 'I want to lose weight'? How much weight do you want to lose, and by when?

Goal: Say you weigh 75 kilos now and it is 1 January, and in three months' time you want to be 5 kilos lighter. So, you would write your goal like this:

> *I weigh 70 kilos by midnight on the 1st of April.*

Or:

> *My goal is to lose 5 kilos and by the 1st of April I am 5 kilos lighter.*

Write your goals down as if you had already achieved them and then work back from there.

The same principle can be applied to the other examples as well:

- 'I want to get fit' – what does that mean? Do you, for example, want to be able to run five kilometres in under 30 minutes in three months' time? Or do you want to be able to complete a circuit within a certain time by a certain date?

- 'I want to tone up' – again, what does it mean? Do you want to reduce your body fat percentage and or increase your muscle mass to a certain number by a certain date?

- 'I want to get stronger' – what would this look like for you? For example, do you want to be able to bench, squat or deadlift a certain weight by a certain date?

Being noticeably clear and specific about what you want will make it easier for you to achieve your goals.

ARE YOU CAPABLE OF ACHIEVING A GOAL?

Absolutely! Just tell your brain what you want and why you want it and see what happens. If we tell our brains what it is that we want, when we lock it in through goal setting, whatever goal we give our subconscious mind, our brain will start finding ways to help us achieve that goal. It will look for the people, organisation, resources, information and opportunities to help us achieve whatever it is that we want.

For example, at the writing of this book my wife and I have a newborn baby – our daughter Rosa. So, when we go to Caneland Shopping Centre with our daughter, guess what we notice? We start noticing all the babies, mums with prams, pregnant women, young families and so on that we did not notice before when our brains were not consumed with the thought and presence of our own little girl.

The same thing happens with goal setting. When we tell our brains what it is that we want and have strong emotional connections towards that image of what we want, our brain then suddenly begins to present us with the opportunities and resources that we need to achieve that goal but couldn't notice before – though they may have been there all along. That is the magical power of goal setting.

Try it and see how this changes your life for the better. Let's work through an example.

What do you want?

Ask yourself: 'What do I want? What is my desire?' Write down 10 things that you want. Let's say three of those things for example are:

1. I want an abundance of energy and vitality.

2. I want to have a body that I am happy with. I want to be able to look in the mirror and be happy with what I see. I want to be happy with my physical appearance.

3. I want to be a great role model for my children and loved ones with the lifestyle that I lead.

Why do you want it?

Again, ask yourself: 'Why do I want what I want? How would this change my life or the lives of others if I get what I want? What impact or difference could I make as a result of getting what I want?' So again, write down the top 10 reasons why you want the top 10 things you have written before. Using the three examples from above, it would look like this:

1. **I WANT an abundance of energy and vitality.**

   WHY? So that I can be more productive at work and still have loads of energy left to run around with my children and entertain my partner when I get home from work.

2. **I WANT to have a body that I am happy with. I want to be able to look in the mirror and be happy with what I see. I want to be happy with my physical appearance.**

   WHY? It will make me feel incredibly good about myself and it will boost my self-esteem and give me the confidence I need to perform at my best.

3. **I WANT to be a great role model for my children and loved ones with the lifestyle that I lead.**

   WHY? My lack of exercise and poor food choices are affecting my children. They are copying my bad examples and I do not want them to think that this is normal. If I do not do something about changing my lifestyle, my children will pass on my bad examples to their own children.

How are you going to achieve what you want?

What information, resources, opportunities, people, and ways are you going to look for to help you achieve your goals? What skills and knowledge would you have to acquire? Depending on the size of the fire under your desire, depending on how big your WHY is, depending on how bad you want it, it will drive you to do whatever it takes to get to your goal.

Let's say for example we are going off the three examples from above; there are a couple of ways that you can achieve all of that. One, you can do it on your own. You can look for information and resources to help you achieve those goals. Or, you can look for people who can help you get there – sometimes sooner than you would on your own. Examples of such people would be a personal trainer, a nutritionist or dietician.

When do you want it?

We live in an age where everything we want has to be achieved yesterday. Everything we want now is at our fingertips. We want instant gratification. If we want to watch a movie or listen to music, we can stream it. If we want to get into a relationship, all we have to do is swipe. We can have a meal delivered to our door in minutes without getting up from the couch. All of these things, while they may seem appealing, cloud our judgment when it comes to being realistic about when important goals such as the three examples mentioned above can or should be achieved. When you turn on the TV today, open a magazine or get on the internet, there are loads of advertisements and information offering quick fixes. *Lose 10 kilos in 10 days. Get chiselled abs in a week.* While these may be enticing to the reader, the truth is they are nothing but quick fixes. And the results do not last – if they are achieved at all.

So, when should you aim to achieve your goal? The answer to this question is that you have to be realistic with yourself and under-stand the things that are important in life take time. They do not just happen overnight. Having this in mind, set deadlines for yourself. If you get to your deadline and you have not achieved your goal, never give up. Move the timeline or deadline. (But, moving the deadline is a last resort, and should only be considered if the other option is to abandon the goal. Otherwise, prioritise meeting your deadlines and sub-deadlines.)

The more you do this, the better you will get at setting deadlines. But first, it is especially important that you give yourself a deadline to achieve your goal by and work hard to make that deadline.

TIME FOR SOME ACTION

Okay! I'm a firm believer that knowledge is only potential power. Applied knowledge is true power. So, here are some actions you can take to help you achieve your goals:

Plan:

- Identify what you want and why you want it.

- Prioritise your goals. Write them down in their order of importance.

- Put in place measures and standards to track your progress.

- Set deadlines and sub-deadlines.

- Identify key obstacles and difficulties that stand between you and your goals.

- Identify knowledge and skills you may need to acquire that will give you the confidence and courage you need to achieve your goals.

- Identify people, groups, organisations and resources to help you achieve your goals.

Action:

- Set your identity and let that identity influence your actions. Who can achieve the goal you want to achieve? Become that person first by taking on that identity. Not at the end. For example, if I am a non-smoker, what does a non-smoker do?

- Write down your goals. Do not just keep them in your head.

- Visualise your goals. Picture them in your mind and write them in places that will make it hard for you to forget them.

- Measure your goals in space and time – *how much* and *by when*.

- Work on your goals daily. What is the one thing you could do today that will help you get closer to your goals?

- Check your expectations. Do not compare yourself to others. Your today might be another person's yesterday.

- Focus on what is working. NOT on what is not working. Focusing on the things that are not working can derail your goal and sabotage your progress.

- Understand that you will not be perfect. There will be stumbles along the way. But remember, it is never how many times you fall that matters. It is how many times you get back up.

- Track and keep a written record of your progress – you cannot manage what you cannot measure.

- Break your goals down into as many smaller parts as possible – the journey of a thousand miles does not only begin with a single step, it is a combination of many single ones.

HOW I HAVE APPLIED GOAL-SETTING

The following four stories will help show how I have applied all the goal-setting lessons I have learned to get to where I am today.

Somewhere to live

Coming from a country that went through 14 years of civil war, being separated from my family at a young age and growing up in refugee camps was horrible. But in the midst of all that, God was good. He kept me alive for a reason and He protected me all the time.

The story of my life would be incomplete if I do not share the important roles that both church and God have played in my life.

Growing up in a refugee camp, there were a lot of bad things that I could have done. I could have done drugs; I could have become a thief; I could have mixed with the wrong crowds. But I found God instead, and I found myself in church, and that helped to shape me into becoming the person that I am today. I remember at the time of receiving salvation, I was homeless. And I remember praying to God and asking him, 'Father, if you are real and you truly saved me, then please show me a sign; please help me with somewhere to live.'

If you are not familiar with the Bible and Christian life, this may sound like an otherworldly story, but asking God for a sign is not unusual. So, when I asked God to help me with a place to live, I trusted and believed that he would. He said in Philippians Chapter 4 verse 19 that he would provide all of my needs according to his riches in glory. I believed, and as God would have it, by word of mouth through my circle of friends, I was introduced to a gentleman named Darlington whom I did not really know at the time other than the fact that I would see him walk past occasionally and stop for a chat with people I knew. As it turned out, Darlington had a vacant one-bedroom apartment. He had recently moved in with his wife and was seeking someone to look after it. Fortunately, that person became me.

Call it perfect timing, luck, chance, whatever you want – I call it the grace of God. I lived in that apartment free of charge until I could afford my own place.

A miracle (continued from step 1)

One of my favourite verses from the Bible is Proverbs 16.9 – it says, 'a man's heart plans his way, but the Lord directs his steps'. As I mentioned earlier in this book, to make life a little easier on myself, I decided to study IT. I could have studied a lot of different things, but of all things I chose to do Information Technology. After I had completed my studies, I got a job at a local internet cafe. Financially, things were a bit better but that was not the only benefit of the job.

Through that job, in a Christian chat room I met Denise Rougier – the incredible woman who helped me come to Australia.

Denise was born in England in 1950 and migrated to Australia in 1955 with her parents. She had a humble upbringing growing up on a farm with her parents and sister, Linda. A mother to two children of her own, Shelley and David, Denise is also a grandmother to nine children – six from Shelley and my three, as I consider her to be my Australian mother.

Denise is a strong believer of Christ. When we first met, we would talk about God all the time and pray for each other and share stories from the Bible. After I received salvation, I wanted to share the good news with others so that they knew what I knew. So, I used to go around with my Pastor Evans Donkor to share the good news. I learned so much from doing that. When Denise and I would talk about God, she was fascinated about how much I could contribute to the conversation. Through those conversations and prayers, one thing led to another, she asked for my story and I told her. And she promised she was going to help me come to Australia. I had never had that kind of conversation before. I prayed that it would happen and here I am today.

While writing this chapter, Denise confessed to me that helping an African child who was an orphan from a war-torn country come over to Australia was something that she had always wanted to do. Many years prior to our meeting, when she received her Australia citizenship, she prayed to God and was frustrated that it was not fair that she could not bring a child over because she was not rich or well off. And then when she finally met me and decided to help, it all seemed impossible. I was an adult; she could not really adopt me. She said many people told her that trying to bring me over was near impossible, but God answered her prayers from many years ago and helped her help me come over.

I came to Australia on a Humanitarian Visa – something that I am forever grateful for and I feel indebted to this country for giving me the opportunity to achieve everything I have today. It is the perfect country for anyone to succeed if they are willing to have a go.

When I first migrated to Australia, things were not as they are today. As I mentioned earlier, years before I even dreamt of coming to Australia, I would tell friends that one day I would leave this continent of Africa and when I do, wherever I go, the ground would shake as a sign that a great man has entered the land. Thinking back now, I laugh because it seems so silly, but it was something I would say all the time!

Funny enough when I landed at Brisbane International Airport on 14 May 2009, the ground did not shake at all. Can you believe it? I thought something was wrong – ha! But let me tell you what happened. I got out of the plane and it was a cool autumn morning. The temperature on my skin and the smell in the air reminded me of how far away from home I had come. I grabbed my bags and asked for directions to the domestic terminal. They pointed me in the way of the air train terminal. There I experienced one of my first and most profound memories of being in Australia. When my son Malachi was born, we were thinking about how we would decorate his room, and so my wife and I decided to put up portraits in his room of some sporting greats who defied the odds as a reminder that no matter where you come from, you can be anything you want to be if you put mind to it. We put up portraits of:

- **Roger Federer** – a young man who was ruled 'unsuitable' for the Swiss Armed Forces to becoming one of the greatest tennis players of all time.

- **Michael Phelps** – a young man who took up swimming as a means to calm his ADHD to becoming the greatest swimmer of all time.

- **Mohammed Ali** – a kid who learned how to box because someone stole his bike to becoming one of the greatest boxers of all time.

- **Michael Jordan** – a high schooler who was not deemed good enough to make his varsity team to becoming the greatest basketball player of all time.

- **Babe Ruth** – a seven-year-old child who was sent to a reformatory orphanage by his parents and became one of the greatest baseball players of all time.

- **George Weah** – a boy who grew up in abject poverty in Liberia (my country of birth) to becoming the only African footballer (soccer player) to win FIFA's Best Player of the World title and now President of the Republic of Liberia.

- We had a portrait of **Jesus Christ**, saviour of the world for anyone who believes.

- We also had **Cathy Freeman** and **Tiger Woods** on the wall.

My wife also asked me to write something that she would put up on the wall. So, I wrote: 'My son, you can be whoever you want to be and achieve anything you want in life if you want it bad enough. When I, your father, first moved here to this country Australia, I could not afford the $2 air train fee from the international terminal to the domestic terminal. Today through hard work and determination I have everything I could ever dream of, including you.'

This was to echo my sentiment that it is not where you come from or where you are today in your life that matters, but where you want to be and how bad you really want to get there.

Yep! I did not have the $2 at the time to pay. Seeing that I was new to the country, the security guard had pity on me and let me through free of charge. I always remember that incident every time I go to Brisbane International Airport. How times have changed. There is even now a free shuttle bus service running people from the international terminal to the domestic terminal and vice versa.

When I got to the domestic terminal, I had to wait nine hours before my connecting flight to Mackay. I had no money and no food. I borrowed someone's phone to let Denise know that I was in

Australia. She tried ringing the airport staff to let them know that I was an immigrant in the country for the first time and that I was transiting for nine hours but had no money for food, and asked if they could help. Australia being the generous country that it is, someone came to help, but by the time they got to me it was about an hour before I boarded my flight to the sugar cane capital of Australia – Mackay. I quickly ate something and then went to my gate.

When I landed in Mackay, Denise and Monique were there to pick me up from the airport. Monique was Denise's grandson Michael's girlfriend. Monique and Michael are now married with a beautiful little boy named Marcus.

Anyway, when we got to the house, I realised that Denise being a pensioner only lived on government payments from fortnight to fortnight. I remember we did not have bath soap in the house, so she gave me her shampoo and said, 'Use this to shower until payday'.

Denise is an incredible woman with an amazing heart. How someone in her position could have helped me come to Australia is a miracle. She is one of my greatest inspirations in life. She is not wealthy; she does not have a job and she is just a pensioner but with a heart that is bigger than most wealthy people in the world. She pleaded on my behalf to the Australian Government that if I came here, I would have a place to stay and not be on the streets. And indeed, I stayed at Denise's house until I could afford to move out.

Denise taught me that you do not need a lot to do a lot. The same inspiration I use in my business today. Starting with absolutely nothing to owning two gyms today.

Against all odds – expanding the gym

In 2017, after eight years of living in Australia, I went back to Africa for the first time to visit. Upon my arrival I was instantly reminded of the hardships and difficulties I was fortunate enough to have left behind. I thought to myself – I am not better than or different to anyone living here in Africa. I just got blessed with the opportunity to move to Australia. If I were still here, I would be just like the people struggling to make ends meet. Going to bed not knowing where the next meal to feed themselves and their families is going to come from. Having qualifications but no jobs. Living among deep corruption. I was also reminded of how fortunate I was to be in Australia, and of all the opportunities I had and the privileges that we sometimes take for granted.

After seeing all the hardship and difficulties and being reminded of all the opportunities I had in Australia, I was inspired to do something with my business. After I had written down my goals for the year for when I returned to Australia, I sat down at the airport and posted this on my social media pages:

> Almost 8 years ago I sat at this boarding gate – Gate 1A at Kotokai International Airport, Accra, Ghana, without an iPhone 6s to do a status update. Social media was not really popular back then. But I had so much hunger in me about things I would do when I got to Australia. That hunger led me to accomplish (in less than 8 years) things that would have otherwise taken me a lifetime.

> Today I cannot say that I have that exact same hunger I had almost 8 years ago, but I know for a fact that I'm definitely a lot hungrier now than I was when I left Australia 2 and half weeks ago.

> It has been great coming back here and meeting family – lots of whom I had not seen since I was a little boy and meeting my nephews and nieces. It has been great being reminded of how life here, is a lot different to what it is in Australia.

> I am not a tourist here, so I did not stay long in a hotel room. It has been humbling not having electricity some nights and taking baths from a bucket and not having running water. And watching people cook from a coal pot and draw water from a well – all things we take for granted and do not think about in Australia. It was great to see my nephew make

dumbbells from cement, a steel pipe, and some empty plastic containers. I remember using makeshift dumbbells like his many years ago.

It has been great eating a lot of African dishes and proudly walking out of any cafe or restaurant that did not sell local food.

Though corruption is still a major cause of poverty across the continent, it has been great to see some improvements and I hope that though slow, change will come – but then again, I am an optimist.

It has been great and I cannot wait to come back here with my family one day but in the meantime, I miss my babies like crazy so I'm really looking forward to getting home and seeing them, feeling them and smelling them again. Sounds weird I know but touch and smell are things that you cannot get from a video call.

Finally, I cannot wait to officially start my working year for 2017! So, I hope you – my clients and future clients – are ready because I am coming at you with everything I have got plus more!!

Thank you, Mama Africa, until next time God bless!

With the above posted to my audience I was ready to tackle 2017 with all the inspiration I was filled with. I was ready.

One of my goals for 2017 was to expand my gym. Now while this seemed like a good idea, the reality was that we did not have the numbers to support that idea. On every account, it seemed like an impossible dream. My business, though we had a gym, was predominantly a one-on-one personal training business. I was selling my hours for dollars. This was okay for a number of years. I loved what I did, and I loved seeing the transformations my clients were getting. So, I did not mind working the ridiculous hours and long days that

I worked. But after my son was born, it was time for me to cut back on those hours.

But spending time with my wife and son presented a huge challenge considering I traded my hours for dollars. After my son was born, for the first time I had to hire an employee to look after the gym when I was not there. Though it seemed like the logical thing to do, for a business whose income was predominantly based on my time, financially it was not viable. Every hour I spent away from the gym, I had to pay someone to be there.

I decided to do something about it. I started looking for ways to scale the business, so it was not so reliant on me. I considered so many options, one of which was to close the gym side of things and just do personal training when I was not with my family, but then I thought that would defeat the purpose of why I decided to open a gym in the first place – to provide a gym environment and experience for the everyday people that was nothing like what they had seen in gyms before. It would also mean that I was still trading hours for dollars. So, for the next two years I ran Muscle Garden at a loss. Mackay was going through a recession at the time, but we were not really affected that much except for the fact that being a father I now had to change my business strategy if I wanted Muscle Garden to still be around.

I remember going to a business course in Melbourne that a friend of mine invited me to attend. The course went for about three days, and after I had left the course and came back to Mackay, a few days later the guy who ran the course rang me to see if I was interested in taking up his mastermind program. He explained how it would help me solve my problem. While it sounded good, I just honestly could not afford the program at the time.

But I was determined to expand the gym and take on bigger overheads. I knew the guy in the shop next to me had his lease running out in August of 2017. (R.I.P. Video Ezy.) My plan was to move in then or shortly after he had moved out. My strategy was to gradually build up the gym membership. So, I started advertising more for gym members. The numbers started to increase little by little. But the number of gym members was one thing. I also needed money to buy new gym equipment. Because I had run the business at a loss for two years in a row, the banks were not going to look at me. My numbers were not good to be considered for a loan. That is when I decided to ask my clients.

It was a big thing for me. I have never done anything like that before. But when you set a goal and lock it in, things start to align to help you achieve that goal. You get the information, resources, and people you need – and even God, or what some people may refer to as the universe – to chip in to help you achieve that goal. I feel like this was the case with some of the equipment I have in my gym today.

Not many people knew my plans to expand the gym. But at the time I was looking for gym equipment and getting quotes for the extra pieces I wanted to add to the gym, a friend of my friend Mick saw on Gumtree that this gym in Brisbane had closed down and they were selling all of their gym equipment. Funny thing is, I do not even remember telling Mick that I was looking for gym equipment to buy. Anyway, Mick's friend had sent him this link and he decided to forward it on to me. When I saw the list of equipment and the price, I could not believe my luck. The whole package cost less than the few pieces I was getting quotes for. I immediately rang the sellers, and after a brief conversation – mainly me bargaining to bring the price down – I immediately paid a deposit on the equipment.

Leverage – help from members

Going to my clients and asking them to help me purchase gym equipment for the expansion of the gym was something that I had not done before and it was definitely way outside of my comfort zone, but if I know one thing about comfort zones, it's that nothing worth having is ever achieved within comfort zones. You have to step outside of your comfort zone, and you have to push the boundaries.

'Why not go out on a limb? Isn't that where the fruit is?'
— Frank Scully

One of the greatest benefits I have found in treating people like human beings is that they will respond to you and give of themselves to you and will even go out of their way to help you when you need them to. I have been blessed to meet some really amazing people through Muscle Garden and I am eternally grateful.

When I had the idea of approaching my clients to see if they would help me get some gym equipment for the expansion, I had no idea how it would go. But I believed that if I did not try, I would not know. I went to my clients with this idea:

Hey Chantel,

You have been training with me for a little while now and I can foresee that you are not planning on leaving soon; if that is the case, I have a deal for you. As you already know, I am planning on expanding the gym, but I have not got enough money to purchase all of the equipment and I cannot go to the banks because we have run at a loss for two years in a row now. This amazing deal just came up on Gumtree. There is a gym down in Brisbane that has closed their doors and they are selling off all of their equipment. I have put a deposit on the equipment, but I need money to pay off the rest. So, here is your deal: if you can prepay some of your personal training sessions, I would give you a $10 per session discount.

Chantel did not hesitate. She asked me how much I needed and paid the funds into my account the next day. She was happy to help me achieve my goal if it meant it would help her achieve hers. And there were many other clients who willingly helped me out. Fortunately, with God's blessings, many things aligned to help me achieve my goal of expanding the gym. Chantel went on to lose 31 kilos in 12 months and completely changed the way she looked. Here are her before and after photos.

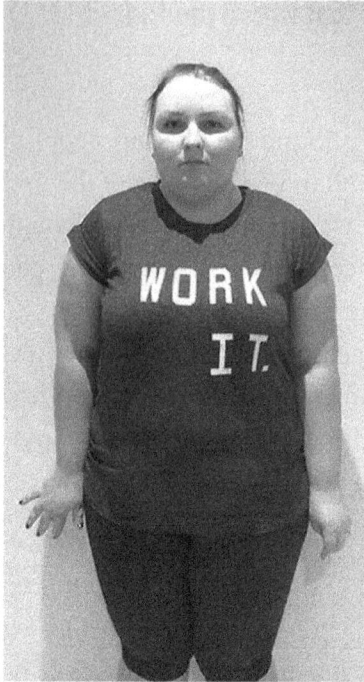

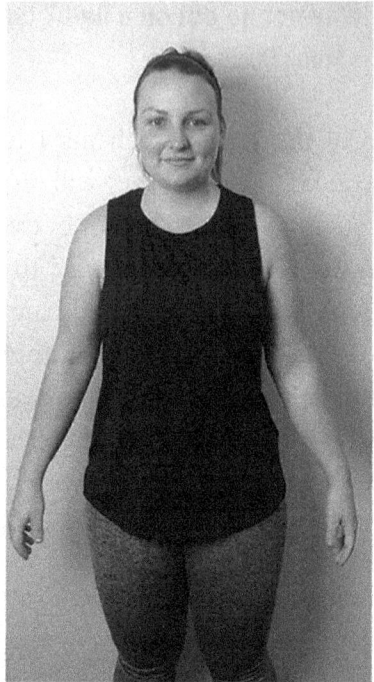

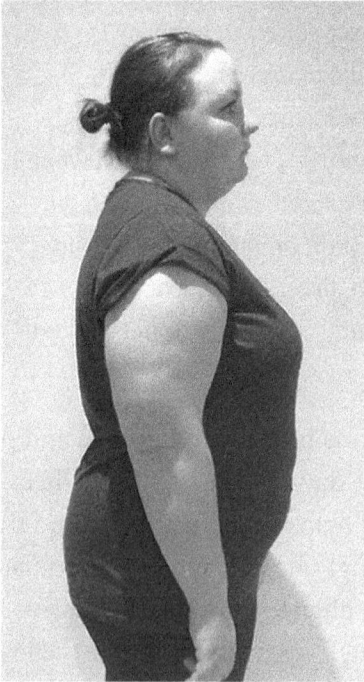

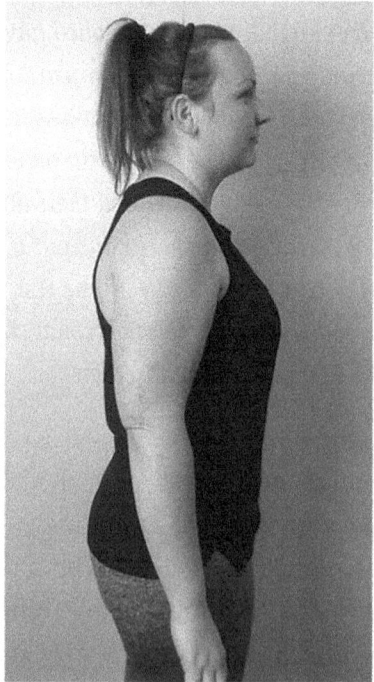

Before and after photos of Chantel

Separation

At the writing of this book, 2017 was by far my hardest year in Australia, and that is saying a lot considering in 2020 we lived through the Coronavirus pandemic lockdowns and I had to shut both of my gyms down.

The year 2017 nearly broke me, but it also made me better and stronger and I am glad to still be here today. I suffered a lot. I learned a lot, and I achieved a lot, in 2017.

I watched my dream turn into my worst nightmare. And without doubt it was an incredibly difficult time for my wife too. When I came back from Africa, my wife and I had some serious disagreements, and as many of you married people would know, marriage is not always easy. As a result of those disagreements and many unresolved issues that came to the surface, my wife and I decided to separate. And since she had moved to Mackay to be with me, she made the decision to move back home to Tweed Heads, 1054.7km from where we lived.

It was extremely hard because we had a son.

I will never forget the day I dropped him off for the first time. I have had some tough times in my life but that was different; that was gut wrenching. It was even harder when I got back to Mackay. I would go to work, and it would feel like my soul had left me. My dream had turned into a nightmare. My wife was not around, and my son was not around anymore. I'm a muscular guy so people would naturally have the perception that I am a strong person, but during those times I was as fragile as I could be. Many days I would go into my office or excuse myself and go the bathroom and cry. Even though I was surrounded by so many of my lovely clients at work, I would go home to an empty house. I felt so lonely and isolated.

And to add to the trauma, I found out that my beloved nephew, whom I had just spent about two weeks hanging out with in Africa, had died. He'd never left my side for the whole two weeks I was there. He came with me everywhere I went. He reminded me every day that, 'Uncle Kay, I am your special bodyguard'. In the midst of what I was going through, when I heard the news of his passing, I was shattered. What hurt even more was that I had plans for him. And he died before I could even start on those plans. He died from something that could have been so easily prevented if he were in Australia.

Anyway, through all the pain and suffering, I never gave up. I never gave up on myself and I never gave up on my goal of expanding the gym. If anything, it inspired me to be better on every level of my life. Working on my business and expanding the gym may have seemed like I was putting my business before my family, but I was not. It was the other way around. If my wife were to move back, I did not want her to move back to the same conditions that we were in. I wanted it to be better. I wanted to be better.

I took my personal development to another level. I read more books, listened to more podcasts and audiobooks, and watched educational videos more than I did in previous years. I have learned and implemented things that have changed my life for the better. I also learned some especially important life lessons.

I do not drink alcohol, so I did not resort to drinking. I ate healthily as always, and I kept up my exercise routine. I climbed a mountain almost every weekend as a reminder that the challenges I faced in my personal life and with the business were just part of the journey, and that if I wanted to get to the summit I had to endure the hardship, the pain and the struggle to get there.

I confided in some close friends and shared my problems and my pains, and it helped having people to talk to.

All these things, along with having a goal, a purpose and something meaningful to work towards, helped me get through.

> **'Happiness comes and goes. But when life is really good and when things are really bad, having meaning gives you something to hold on to.'** – Emily Esfahani Smith

We expanded Muscle Garden from a 155-square-metre gym to a 326-square-metre 24/7 state-of-the-art fitness facility. And I got to live my dream again. After eight painful months, my wife moved back home.

If I had given up on myself and my family, if I had abused my body with alcohol, eaten poorly, given up on exercise and was filled with hate and anger and had no meaning and no goals to chase, this would not have been possible. But I did not want my son growing up between two homes. This was not the life I envisioned for him, and it certainly was not what I wanted for him. I lost my dad at a young age, so I wanted to be there for my son. I never gave up. I did not want a divorce. It was not an option when I decided to get married. I loved my wife and I wanted our family to grow and I wanted to grow old with her.

Through all the struggles, one thing I was reminded of is that the best does not always happen in life, but you can always make the best out of what does happen. I am grateful to all those who were there for me during my darkest moments. And I am thankful to all those who helped make my brightest moments possible.

Never give up. Always look back on your life. It was the hardest moments that made you who you are.

STEP 3

INCLUDE GOOD
NUTRITION
FOR A HEALTHY AND
HAPPY LIFE

According to the World Health Organization, nutrition is defined as the intake of food, considered in relation to the body's dietary needs. Good nutrition – an adequate, well-balanced diet – combined with regular physical activity is a cornerstone of good health. Poor nutrition can lead to reduced immunity, increased susceptibility to disease, impaired physical and mental development, and reduced productivity.

Simply, nutrition is the process by which we intake and utilise food substances for energy, sustenance, health, and growth of our body. Unfortunately, some food can have the opposite effect on our body, causing sickness and sometimes death.

So what *is* a nutrient?

A nutrient is a component of food that provides nourishment for our body; examples are carbohydrates, fats, proteins, vitamins, minerals, fibre and water.

There are two types of nutrients:

- *Macronutrients* are nutrients our body needs in relatively large quantities.

- *Micronutrients* are nutrients our body needs in relatively smaller quantities.

Macronutrients can be further broken down into energy-producing macronutrients – such as carbohydrates, fats and proteins – and non-energy-producing macronutrients – such as fibre and water. Let's have a look at some of the most important nutrients in our diet.

Carbohydrates (4 calories per gram)

When you hear the word 'carbohydrates' – or 'carbs' for short – what are the first few things that come to your mind? You may be thinking rice, bread, pasta, potatoes, and you would be right. But carbs are not just found in those food items. They are also present in fruits and vegetables, as well as grains and sugary foods.

Carbs can simply be defined as:

- simple sugars – monosaccharide (glucose, fructose, galactose)
- two sugar molecules – disaccharides (sucrose, lactose, maltose)
- long chains of sugar molecules – polysaccharides (starch, cellulose, glycogen).

The glycaemic index helps us understand how the carbs we eat affect our blood sugar level. It is defined as the number associated with the carbohydrates in a particular type of food that indicates the effect of these carbohydrates on a person's blood sugar level. Foods are classified into low-GI, medium-GI or high-GI on the glycaemic index. A low-GI food will cause blood sugar levels to increase more slowly and steadily, and a high-GI food causes a more rapid rise in blood sugar levels.

Simple sugars or high-GI foods – such as the obvious: soft drinks, cakes, chocolates, ice cream, biscuits, fruit juice – and the not so obvious: white bread, white rice, potatoes, cereals – are easily digested and rapidly release glucose into the blood stream, which causes a huge spike in blood sugar levels. This may be suitable for energy recovery after a workout, although if weight loss is your goal, it will be wise to be very mindful of how much of this is consumed. This is also suitable for a person experiencing low blood sugar levels.

Complex sugars or low-GI foods – such as most vegetables, most fruits, rolled oats, beans, whole wheat, cashews, small seeds (sunflower, flax, pumpkin, sesame, poppy, hemp), brown rice, sweet potatoes, mushrooms, chilli – slowly and steadily release glucose into the blood stream, which helps to regulate blood sugar levels and avoid huge insulin spikes (something we will talk about later in this step). For example: fruit juice might be high-GI but the fruit itself is low-GI; the difference between the two is fibre. Fibre is present in the fruit and not in the juice.

Over 40% of your energy intake is going to come from carbs. So, to avoid the confusion of which carbs are the right or wrong ones, it is best to check the glycemic index to find out which carbs are low-GI, medium-GI or high-GI foods. There are some examples in the table below.

Classification	GI range	Examples
Low GI	55 or less	fructose, most beans, most small seeds (like sunflower seeds, flax seeds, pumpkin seeds, sesame seeds, etc), walnuts, cashews, wheat, millet, oat, rye, rice, barley, vegetables, sweet fruits (like peaches, strawberries, mangos), mushrooms, chilli
Medium GI	56–69	white sugar, wheat, pita bread, basmati rice, grape juice, raisins, prunes, cranberry juice, ice cream, banana, sweet potato
High GI	70 and above	glucose, high fructose corn syrup, white bread, white rice, most breakfast cereals, white potato

Fats (9 calories per gram)

Some people cringe when they hear the words 'fat' or 'fatty food', and that's because according to what they have heard, fat leads to being overweight or obesity and heart disease. While there is truth in that, fat is actually essential in our diet.

Fats serve many functions in our body. They lubricate our joints, preserve brain health, and help our organs produce hormones. They also assist in the absorption of certain vitamins, reduce inflammation, help to prevent very dry skin and are a source of energy. This being said, diets that are high in fats, especially saturated fats, are associated with weight gain and heart disease.

There are different types of fats, and some fats are healthier than others:

- **Saturated fats** – eating large amounts of saturated fats can increase your risk of heart disease and high blood cholesterol levels. Saturated fats can be found in foods such as fatty cuts of beef, pork, lamb and chicken (especially chicken skin), processed meats like salami, bacon and chorizo, coconut milk and cream, hot chips, pizza, hamburgers, potato chips, savoury crackers, pies and sausage rolls.

The ketogenic diet believes this to be false, and proposes that eating animal fats and fatty food is actually good for the body and poses no risk of heart disease. Given the effects these food items have on the body, they are not something I would recommend as a major part of a sustainable diet.

- **Unsaturated fats** – these do the opposite of saturated fats and they play an important role in a healthy diet. They help to reduce the risk of heart disease and cholesterol levels, along with having other health benefits. There are two types of unsaturated fats:
    - *Polyunsaturated fats:* omega-3 fatty acids, which are found in fish, especially oily fish like mackerel and salmon; omega-6 fatty acids, which are found in oils such as flaxseed oils and hempseed oils.
    - *Monounsaturated fats:* which are found in avocadoes, olive oil and some nuts, including almonds and cashews.

- **Cholesterol** – this is a substance made in our body by the liver. It can also be created by plants, and is found in food like meat and dairy products. Though cholesterol has a negative association, it plays a particularly important role in: the production of hormones such as oestrogen and testosterone; creation and maintenance of cell membranes; bile acid production in the liver, which aids with digestion; and it also helps in the creation of vitamin D.

It's useful to know that not all cholesterols are good. There are two types of cholesterols: LDL (low density lipoproteins) and HDL (high density lipoproteins). Lipoproteins are compounds made of fats and proteins, which carry cholesterol throughout the body in the blood.

LDLs are the 'bad' cholesterols. Too much LDLs in the blood can clog up arteries, cause blood clots and are known to cause heart attacks or strokes. It is recommended to keep LDLs levels low, ideally below 2 millimole per litre (mmol/L) to avoid the aforementioned conditions. A millimole is one-thousandth of a mole. Mmol/L gives the molarity, which is the number of molecules of a substance (in this case blood sugar level) within a specified volume, in this case one litre.

HDLs are considered the 'good' cholesterol. They help to take LDLs out of the blood stream back to the liver, where they are broken down and excreted out of the body through faeces.

What is a healthy cholesterol level? According to Bupa Australia, below are the Australian guidelines for fasting blood cholesterol levels to help reduce your risk of developing cardiovascular disease.

Total cholesterol	Below 4.0 mmol/L
LDL cholesterol	Below 2.0 mmol/L
HDL cholesterol	Above 1.0 mmol/L

Protein (4 calories per gram)

The third of our macronutrients is an essential component of our muscle, skin, and bones. As you would have noticed above, both proteins and carbohydrates contribute the same number of calories per gram (4 calories) while fats contribute 9 calories per gram.

There are 20 amino acids – organic compounds found in nature – which combine to form proteins. When protein is broken down into amino acids, the liver absorbs what it needs through digestion and the rest circulates to the body's cells, which the cells use for the functions of making enzymes, membranes, muscle proteins, hormones and so on. Some amino acids are essential, which means they need to be consumed, and other amino acids are non-essential because the body can produce them.

Meat, eggs, fish, milk, soy, tofu, legumes, beans, nuts, and some cereals are sources of proteins. But choose your protein wisely, as not all proteins are created equal. A piece of steak may be a good source of protein, but it can also be a source of saturated fats. Processed meats such as sausages, salami, ham, bacon and chorizo have been linked to increased risk of type 2 diabetes, cardiovascular disease and some cancers.

A common misconception is that protein builds muscles. While protein is a building block of muscles and helps with growth and repair of muscles, protein on its own without exercise does not build muscles. Muscle fibres have to contract and experience some microscopic tears for proteins to help them grow.

Another misconception that needs to be clarified is that more protein equals more muscles. More protein does not equal more muscles. There is a recommended daily intake of protein that is required by our body that is 10% to 35%. True, all protein comes from our diet. I am referring to diets that are heavy on protein and less on everything irrespective of what the recommended daily intake is. All the macronutrients we consume in a day should amount to 100% of our energy consumption within their daily recommended guidelines, otherwise we are not consuming a balanced diet. To build muscle, only one gram of protein per kilogram of body weight is recommended. Excess protein has been proven to cause weight gain, dehydration, nutrient deficiencies, kidney problems and more.

Fibre

Fibre is one of two macronutrients that do not provide energy. The other one is water. Our body needs these two in large quantities just like carbs, fats and proteins.

Fibre is mostly carbohydrate, but because it's not easily absorbed into the body, most of its sugar and starches do not get into the blood stream. Fibre can also be referred to as 'roughage', the indigestible part of plant foods that travels through our digestive system, absorbing water along the way, and helps to ease bowel movements. Fibre has a lot of health benefits, including reducing the risk of type

2 diabetes and cardiovascular disease. Fibre is mostly found in vegetables, fruits, grains, seeds and legumes.

There are two types of fibre: soluble and insoluble. Soluble fibre dissolves in water and changes its form as it goes through the digestive tract, where it is fermented by bacteria. Examples of soluble fibre include oranges, flax seeds, Brussels sprouts, oats, and beans (pinto, kidney, and black beans), broccoli, zucchini, apples, and grapes. Among other functions, soluble fibre helps to reduce cholesterol levels, especially the 'bad' LDL cholesterols.

Insoluble fibre does not dissolve in water and it does not change its form as it goes through the digestive track, and bacteria in the colon can also ferment it. Dark leafy greens, root vegetables and fruit skins are all examples of insoluble fibre. Insoluble fibre helps with frequent bowel movements and prevents constipation.

Water

Water is the second macronutrient that does not provide energy, which means water has zero calories. About 60% to 70% of our body is water. And our body uses water in all of its cells for vital functions. The benefits of water include:

- it keeps our joints cushioned
- it helps our brains to function properly
- it's a natural remedy for headaches
- it helps with weight management
- it removes wastes and toxins from the body through perspiration, urination and defecation
- it keeps us hydrated and regulates our body temperature
- it prevents cramps and sprains
- it relieves fatigue and improves our mood
- it improves our performance during exercise
- it helps to moisten the air we breathe.

Because we lose water through a lot of bodily functions such as sweating, breathing and digestion, it is vital that we replenish the water we lose by drinking fluids and eating foods rich in water. For example, my favourite fruit is watermelon (nod if that is your favourite fruit too).

Since our body is almost 70% water and water is so vital to our existence, how much of it do you need? There is no 'one cap fits all' rule to how much water is required by an individual. This varies from one person to another, and it also depends on other factors such as the climate you live in (cold, hot or humid), your level of physical activity (low, moderate or high), your health (well or unwell) and the type of work that you do. For example, someone working in a shed in Queensland during summer will require more water than an office worker who sits behind a desk for most of their day.

Not drinking enough water is not good and can lead to dehydration. On the flip side, too much water is also not good and can cause hyponatremia or water intoxication, which is basically drinking too much water within a short period of time. This can cause the salts or sodium in your body to drop too low, and it can sometimes be fatal.

If you are not sure of how much water you should drink, the simplest tool to use is to check your urine colour to see if it is too yellow, light yellow or too clear.

Vitamins

Vitamins are micronutrients – organic compounds that our body requires in smaller amounts for the proper functioning of our metabolism. They cannot be synthesised (produced) by our body, either at all or in sufficient quantities, so they must be obtained from our diets. Like fibre and water, vitamins provide no energy, but they play a vital role in how we function. For example, a deficiency in vitamin B12 may lead to an immediate feeling of tiredness and impair your ability to make healthy red blood cells. Lack of vitamin B12 can cause pernicious anaemia and brain damage, which can lead to death.

Vitamins are classified either as those that can be dissolved in water – water-soluble vitamins – or those that can be dissolved in fat – fat-soluble vitamins.

There are nine water-soluble vitamins (eight different types of vitamin B, and vitamin C) and there are four fat-soluble vitamins (A, D, E and K).

Because water-soluble vitamins are quickly eliminated through our urine and are not stored easily, they need to be consumed more frequently.

Our body absorbs fat-soluble vitamins through the intestines with the help of fats. They are more likely to build up in the body because they are harder to get rid of quickly. Too much build up of vitamins can lead to a condition called hypervitaminosis – abnormally high storage levels of vitamins – which can lead to toxic symptoms.

On the following pages is a table of vitamins and their many different roles and functions, as well as their sources.

Minerals

Like vitamins, minerals are micronutrients that our body requires in smaller quantities. They do not provide energy either, but are also very essential to how our body functions. Minerals are produced in the soil and cannot be made by living organisms. Plants get their minerals from the soil. Most of the minerals in our diet come from eating plants and animals or from drinking water. Like vitamins, essential fatty acids and essential amino acids, minerals are a group of essential nutrients that our body needs to perform functions necessary for life.

There are five major minerals in the human body: calcium, magnesium, phosphorus, potassium and sodium. The rest are called 'trace elements', and those with specific biomechanical functions in our body are: sulphur, iron, chlorine, cobalt, copper, zinc, manganese, molybdenum, iodine, and selenium.

Following is a table of dietary elements – their functions and sources.

Fat-soluble vitamins

Vitamin	Deficiency	Overdose	Food sources
Vitamin A Retinol	Night blindness (poor vision at night or in dimly lit environments)	Hypervitaminosis A (changes to vision and skin, bone pain and possible liver damage and pressure on the brain)	Milk, soy milk, fish, spinach, pumpkin, carrots, leafy vegetables, ripe yellow fruits, liver
Vitamin D Cholecalciferol	Rickets and osteomalacia (softening and weakening of bones in children)	Hypervitaminosis D (rare but potentially serious). Can cause abnormally high levels of calcium in the blood which can affect bones, tissues and other organs. High blood pressure, bone loss and kidney problems can result if not treated.	Eggs, liver, sardines, shiitake mushroom, lichen
Vitamin E tocopherols	Very rare; mild hemolytic anaemia in newborn infants, sterility in males and miscarriage in females	Likely to increase chances of congestive heart failure	Nuts and seeds and many fruits and vegetables
Vitamin K phylloquinone	Bleeding diathesis (unusual susceptibility to bleeding)	Reduced anticoagulation effect of warfarin	Egg yolks, liver, leafy green vegetables such as spinach

Water-soluble vitamins

Vitamin	Deficiency	Overdose	Food sources
Vitamin B1 Thiamine	Beriberi	Relaxed muscle and drowsiness	Eggs, liver, pork, potatoes, oatmeal, brown rice, vegetables
Vitamin B2 Riboflavin	Ariboflavinosis (sores on the mouth)		Bananas, green beans, asparagus, dairy products, popcorn
Vitamin B3 Niacin	Pellagra (diarrhoea, dementia, swollen skin, sores in the mouth)	Liver damage	Tree nuts, mushroom, many vegetables, eggs, fish, meat
Vitamin B5 Pantothenic acid	Paresthesia ('pins-and-needles' sensation, prickling or tingling)	Possible nausea and heartburn, diarrhoea	Broccoli, avocado, meat
Vitamin B6 Pyridoxine	Anaemia	Proprioception impairment (balance issues like not being able to stand on one foot, uncoordinated movement like inability to walk in a straight line)	Bananas, tree nuts, vegetables, meat

Vitamin	Deficiency	Overdose	Food sources
Vitamin B7 Biotin	Dermatitis (skin conditions like itchy, dry skin or rash, eczema and dandruff are examples)		Leafy green vegetables, peanuts, liver raw egg yolk
Vitamin B9 Folates	Megaloblastic anaemia and deficiency during pregnancy is associated with birth defects, such as neural tube defects – most common examples are spina bifida (fetal spinal doesn't close completely) and anencephaly (the brain and skull do not develop) which usually results in stillbirth or death shortly after birth	May mask symptoms of vitamin B12 deficiency	Liver, leafy vegetables, pasta, bread, cereal
Vitamin B12 Cyanocobalamin	Pernicious anaemia (weakened stomach lining, autoimmune condition)	None proven	Beef, poultry, fish
Vitamin C Ascorbic acid	Scurvy	None known	Citrus fruits and vegetables, liver

Dietary elements and their functions and sources

Dietary element	Major mineral/ trace elements	Function	Food sources
Calcium	Major mineral	To maintain strong bones, help muscles to move and many other important functions in the body	Dairy products, eggs, canned fish with bones (salmon, sardines), green leafy vegetables, nuts, seeds, tofu, thyme, oregano, dill, cinnamon
Magnesium	Major mineral	Keeps heartbeat steady, helps bones remain strong and helps to adjust blood glucose levels; also aids in the production of energy and protein	Spinach, legumes, nuts, seeds, wholegrains, peanut butter, avocado
Potassium	Major mineral	Helps with muscle contraction and nerve signals; helps to reduce blood pressure and water retention, regulate fluid balance and prevent osteoporosis and kidney stones	Sweet potato, tomato, potato, beans, lentils, dairy products, seafood, banana, prune, carrot, orange
Phosphorus	Major mineral	Formation of bones and teeth. Helps with how the body uses carbohydrates and fats. Helps in the production of protein for the growth, repair and maintenance of cells and tissues.	Red meat, dairy foods, fish, poultry, bread, rice, oats

Dietary element	Major mineral/ trace elements	Function	Food sources
Sodium	Major mineral	Helps maintain the balance of water in and around our cells and important for proper muscle and nerve function	Table salt (sodium chloride, the main source), sea vegetables, milk, and spinach.
Chlorine	Trace elements	Production of hydrochloric acid in the stomach; helps keep the amount of fluid inside and outside of our cells in balance	Table salt (sodium chloride) is the main dietary source.
Chromium	Trace elements	Helps to break down fats and carbohydrates; important for brain function and other body processes	Broccoli, red grape juice, meat, wholegrain products
Cobalt	Trace elements	Needed for making red blood cells	Vitamin B12, animal and animal-sourced foods
Copper	Trace elements	With iron, helps the body form red blood cells. Also helps keep blood vessels, bones, nerves and immune system healthy; aids in absorption of iron.	Liver, seafood, oysters, nuts, seeds; some wholegrains, legumes

Dietary element	Major mineral/ trace elements	Function	Food sources
Iodine	Trace elements	To make thyroid hormones which control the body's metabolism and many other important functions like proper bone and brain development during pregnancy and infancy	Seaweed, grains, eggs, iodised salt
Manganese	Trace elements	Helps with protein and amino acid digestion and utilisation and the metabolism of cholesterol and carbohydrates	Grains, legumes, seeds, nuts, leafy vegetables, tea, coffee
Molybdenum	Trace elements	Helps break down toxic substances that enter the body and prevent toxins from building up in the body	Legumes, wholegrains, nuts
Selenium	Trace elements	Helps our body make antioxidant enzymes – a type of special proteins which play a role in preventing cell damage	Brazil nuts, seafoods, organ meats, meats, grains, dairy products, eggs
Zinc	Trace elements	Needed for the body's immune system to function properly. Helps with cell division, cell growth, wound healing, and breaking down of carbohydrates. Also needed for the senses of smell and taste.	Oysters, red meat, poultry, nuts, wholegrains, dairy products

HOW SUGAR AFFECTS YOUR BODY

Before we delve into what sugar does to your body, let us first identify what these sugars are. While it's true that you may not sit down and consume 10 teaspoons of sugar, you could be unknowingly doing so in the foods you eat or beverages you drink. Let's take, for example, a simple can of coke: this contains 39 grams of sugar, which is a little over nine teaspoons of sugar. For a male, 39 grams of sugar is more than the daily recommended intake of sugar, being 38 grams. So just by drinking one can of coke you are already over the limit, and you would have consumed close to 10 teaspoons of sugar in just one beverage.

As briefly mentioned earlier in this step under carbohydrates, 'sugar' can be another word for carbohydrates.

Monosaccharide (glucose, fructose, galactose) – often referred to as simple sugars – is a single sugar molecule found in foods such as:

- desserts, cakes, lollies, whipped cream, ice cream, chocolate, chocolate milk, and flavoured yogurt

- sugary drinks like soft drinks, fruit juice, energy drinks, sweetened ice tea, sweetened coffee, smoothies, milkshakes, and alcohol

- jams, jellies, dried fruits, canned fruits, and sauces like barbecue and tomato sauces

- ingredients such as high-fructose corn syrup, molasses, maple syrup, and agave.

Disaccharides (sucrose, lactose, maltose) are two sugar molecules or two monosaccharide that combine to form disaccharides, which can be found in foods such as:

- white sugar, brown sugar, powdered sugar, sugar cane, cane sugar, and raw sugar

- milk, cheese, chocolate, infant formulas, and pudding

- bread products, cereal, energy bars, and candies.

Polysaccharides (starch, cellulose, glycogen) are long chains of sugar and can be found in foods such as:

- pasta, rice, and French fries

- cookies and cakes

- pizzas and bread

- commercial cereals

- corn.

The various examples used above should be consumed with caution, avoided, or minimised depending on what your weight management goals are.

Sugars like glucose help to keep us alive. Our body uses sugar for fuel, and it is vital to our existence. But too much of the examples above can have detrimental effects on our health.

So now that we have an idea of what foods contribute to the sugars in our body, let's get into how our body processes sugar and how it affects us.

How your body processes energy

The pancreas is an organ in our body, and it plays a major role in converting the food we eat into fuel for our body's cells. It has two main functions: *exocrine* function, which helps with digestion, and an *endocrine* function, which helps to regulate blood sugar levels.

Exocrine function

The pancreas has exocrine glands, which release enzymes like trypsin and chymotrypsin to help digest proteins, amylase to help digest carbohydrates, and lipase to help break down fats.

Endocrine function

The pancreas consists of islet cells that create and release two important hormones: insulin – which helps to lower blood sugar levels; and glucagon – which helps to raise blood sugar levels. Having proper blood sugar levels is vital to the functioning of key organs like our liver, brain, and kidneys.

Insulin

In addition to regulating blood sugar levels, insulin also helps to regulate how our body uses and stores fat. Many of the cells in our body rely on insulin to take glucose from the blood for energy. Insulin signals the liver, muscle, and fat cells to take up glucose from the blood for energy. When there is an adequate amount of energy in our body, insulin again signals the liver to take up glucose and store it as glycogen. The liver can store about 5% to 6% of its mass as glycogen.

Simply put, insulin helps our muscle and fat cells absorb the energy we need to function, and because there is only so much that we need, it also helps us store some of that energy as glycogen and it turns any remaining glucose in the blood into saturated body fat.

When you consume simple sugars or high-GI foods, glucose is easily digested and rapidly released into the blood stream. Consuming excess sugar and fats from these foods can lead to weight gain. When you carry too much fat tissue, especially around your waist, your body's cells can become insulin resistant. When your cells cannot utilise insulin properly, your pancreas mistakes this for the need for more insulin so it releases more. Eventually, your pancreas wears out and stops producing enough insulin to help control your blood sugar levels, and this can lead to diabetes, a condition characterised by high blood sugar levels. This is very important to know, and if you remember anything from this step, let it be this.

WHAT IS YOUR RELATIONSHIP WITH FOOD?

Your relationship with food is the difference between you achieving your healthy weight management goals and not. Would you say you have a healthy relationship with food or a not-so-healthy one? What food do you find yourself thinking about most of the time?

And is it a healthy food or something you eat to relieve stress or satisfy your cravings, even though it may not be a healthy choice? Identifying your relationship with food and those food items that taste good in your mouth but are not so good for your body will help you make changes to achieve your health, fitness, and weight goals. As discussed earlier in this step, food is a source of nutrition, energy, and sustenance for the growth and repair of our body, and it should be seen as such. Not as something to be used for stress relief or to be avoided.

Who is in control – you or the food?

Who is in control? Ask yourself: is it you or a particular food item? What is the food that controls you – the one that blinds your judgment and weakens your willpower so that when you see it, you cannot help but to bow at its mercy and have it? It is good to know who is in control, because when you are in control, you can choose to have a food item – whether it is good or not – because you want to have it and not because you feel powerless in front of it. But achieving that kind of willpower where you have the ability to choose and be able to say yes or no to food does not come overnight; it is something that is developed over time.

When the food is in control, especially if it is not contributing to your health in a good way, then there are steps you can take to manage this disorder:

1. **Out of sight, out of mind:** The first thing you can do is to keep the food item out of sight. If you find that this food item or items own you, it is probably not a good thing to have them in your kitchen. This may not be easy to start with, but it's the first step to developing your willpower and taking back control over what you eat. I say 'willpower', but it is more like designing your environment so you don't have to rely on your willpower as to whether to eat or not to eat that particular food that may not be good for you.

2. **Get support:** Surround yourself with people who may be on the same journey as you; people who want to see you do well and not judge you because you are taking steps to improve your health or your eating habits. If you are constantly surrounded by people who eat unhealthily, if you do not have the willpower, this may sabotage your efforts. So, surround yourself with people who will support your habits. Another thing you can do is to form an accountability group with likeminded people who are on the same journey as you, and keep each other accountable and hold each other to a high standard as well as keeping track of your progress.

3. **Plan your day:** One way to prepare yourself to avoid having to eat food that is not good for you is to plan your day. Map out all of your meals for the day. A good plan should include five to six small meals per day, including healthy snacks like fruits and vegetables as well as nuts, seeds and the like that are spread out across the whole day, to avoid overeating and making rash and unhealthy decisions. And even better than having a plan for a day is having a weekly plan. Later on in this step I will give you a simple plan that you can follow to help you reach your health, fitness, and weight management goals.

4. **There is a better way to relieve stress:** Eating may relieve stress, but it is only for the short term. Consider the long-term consequences like weight gain, which poses a number of other health-related problems, before going down this path. Exercise, meditation, yoga, and massage are all great ways that you can relieve stress with proven long-term health benefits.

5. **Get professional help:** If you find you cannot gain back control over what you eat then it may be best to seek some professional help. Talking to a psychologist who works in the area of food disorders may be of help. Seeing a dietician or nutritionist may also prove valuable.

IS 'COUNTING CALORIES' A GOOD IDEA?

I personally do not count calories, and if I did have the time and energy to measure and count every single calorie from every food item I ate, I would probably volunteer that time to charity. My point is, it's too much work and hassle that is not really necessary, unless you are a bodybuilder preparing for a competition or someone on a strict diet to lose weight with a calorie deficit.

Another reason why I do not count calories is because the idea of counting calories can make you lose sight of the nutritional value of some foods simply because they may be high in calories. For example, a medium-size apple is about 95 calories. A mini Mars Bar has 81 calories.

Though I would not recommend counting the calories for every single meal you eat, it is good to be aware of how many calories your body is burning per day and how many you should be having per day. Being aware of these numbers will help you make informed decisions about the nutrition your body needs. One point I always like to stress is that food is for the nourishment, sustenance, growth, and repair of our body. We should not just put food in our mouths for the sake of doing so. I encourage you to ask yourself before putting food in your mouth: is this for the nourishment of my body? What is this going to do for me? What impact is it going to have on my health? When you are clear on the answers to these questions, you will not just eat for the sake of eating. You will be eating and drinking for the nourishment, sustenance, growth, and repair of your body, and this is particularly important because food is medicine. Food has such a huge impact on how we function. It impacts our weight, mood, sleep, energy levels, health, and productivity.

Basal metabolic rate

Your basal metabolic rate (BMR) is the number of calories your body burns while it is at rest. Having an idea of this number will help you determine how many calories you should be having per day.

There are some clinical tests you can do to obtain this number, and there are also machines like the InBody Scanner that can be used to give you close enough numbers about your body. Alternatives to these machines are simple apps you can download to give you some numbers for yourself based on averages. One app to download is a BMR calculator, or you could simply type into Google BMR calculator and it will give you a number of options to choose from.

A good BMR calculator will consider personal factors such as your age, sex, height, and weight. For example, a 45-year-old female who is 165cm tall and weighs 68kg will have a BMR of 1328 calories per day, while a male of the same age with a height of 178cm and weight of 85kg will have a BMR of 1745 calories per day.

To then calculate an estimated number of calories you burn per day, an equation multiplies your BMR by a factor that is based on how active you are. So, again, for example a male with a BMR of 1745 calories per day who exercises lightly for about one to three days per week would burn about 2400 calories per day, while our female example with a BMR of 1328 calories per day, who exercises moderately for about three to five days per week, would burn about 2059 calories per day.

Again, these are just averages. To get more accurate and personalised results I advise that you get a proper scan done, such as a DXA (dual-energy X-ray absorptiometry) scan or an InBody Scan, or something similar.

Using daily energy expenditure to lose, gain or maintain weight

When it comes to losing weight, my advice is to aim for about 500 grams to one kilogram per week. Any more than that and you run into the risk of losing muscle mass and water. Having more muscle mass increases your metabolism, which helps you to burn more calories while your body is at rest. With less muscle mass you burn fewer calories, making weight loss slow and difficult.

To average a weight loss of about 500 grams to one kilogram per week, you would need a caloric deficit of about 3500 to 7000 calories per week or 500 to 1000 calories per day. To gain weight you would apply the same numbers in reverse, and to maintain, you would aim to consume about the same number of calories you burn per day.

> **'When you start eating food without labels, you no longer need to count calories.'** – Amanda Kraft

While there is some truth to the quote above, it would be nearly impossible to only consume foods without labels these days without restricting yourself to just one or two ingredients. Nearly everything we eat today comes with a label, even the healthy stuff.

If you find that counting calories helps to keep you accountable and on track and it seems to be working for you, then by all means continue to do so. As a matter of fact, if weight loss is your goal then counting calories with a caloric deficit is my recommendation. But if you are like me and you think it's too much effort for something that is not really necessary, I still recommend that it is a good idea to be aware of what your numbers are roughly, so that you can make your food choices based around those numbers. Personally, when I am training to put on more muscle mass, my plate size is different to, say, when I am training for a marathon. Though I do not count calories, I am aware of how many calories I burn per day, so I adjust accordingly based on my goal – whether to lose, gain or maintain weight.

HOW AND WHY TO EAT HEALTHILY

Simply put, eating healthily is basically eating a balanced diet – a diet that consists of all the macronutrients (carbohydrates, fats, and proteins; fibre and water) and micronutrients (vitamins and minerals). In a balanced diet, your daily calorie intake should comprise: carbohydrates 45% to 65%, fats 20% to 35%, and proteins 10% to 35%.

So, for example, a balanced diet for me would resemble something like this: carbs 51%, fats 23%, and proteins 26%.

Eating healthily means eating foods that are rich in nutrients, like fruits, vegetables, and nuts, and avoiding processed foods, fast foods, and foods that are high in sugar. It means limiting your alcohol consumption. It also means that you do not just eat for the sake of eating, but you eat and drink for the nourishment, sustenance, growth, and repair of your body.

It also means setting good examples for your loved ones to follow. Eating unhealthily affects your mood, your sleep, energy levels, weight, your productivity at work, and your health in general. And it can also lead to a host of problems like type 2 diabetes, being overweight or obese, heart disease and stroke, some cancers, high cholesterol, high blood pressure, osteoporosis, depression, anxiety, and eating disorders.

Eating healthily has a range of benefits that go way beyond what you could imagine. By eating a healthy diet, you can turn your whole life around. Here are some examples of things that will happen to you as a result of eating healthily:

- Your energy levels will improve – you won't feel as tired or drowsy. You will be more productive at work and will have enough energy to play with your children and entertain your partner when you get home from work.

- You will sleep better at night and feel refreshed and rejuvenated to handle the day ahead.

- Your mood will improve dramatically, and this will help you handle stress better.

- It will help you manage your weight. If weight loss is your goal, eating healthily will help you lose weight and limit your chances of being overweight or obese. When it comes to losing weight, about 80% of weight loss comes down to what you put in your mouth.

- It will improve almost every aspect of your health.
- It will help you set good examples for your loved ones to follow, and also help build the foundation for healthy growth and development as well as learning for children.

Make it a priority to eat healthily because your quality of life depends on it. As the great American president Abraham Lincoln once said: 'And in the end, it's not the years in your life that count; it's the life in your years.'

THE FIVE FOOD GROUPS

For a healthy and balanced diet, it is recommended that we consume foods from different food groups. On the following page is the Australian Guide to Healthy Eating, a food selection guide that visually represents the proportion of the five food groups recommended for consumption each day.

The Australian Guide to Healthy Eating

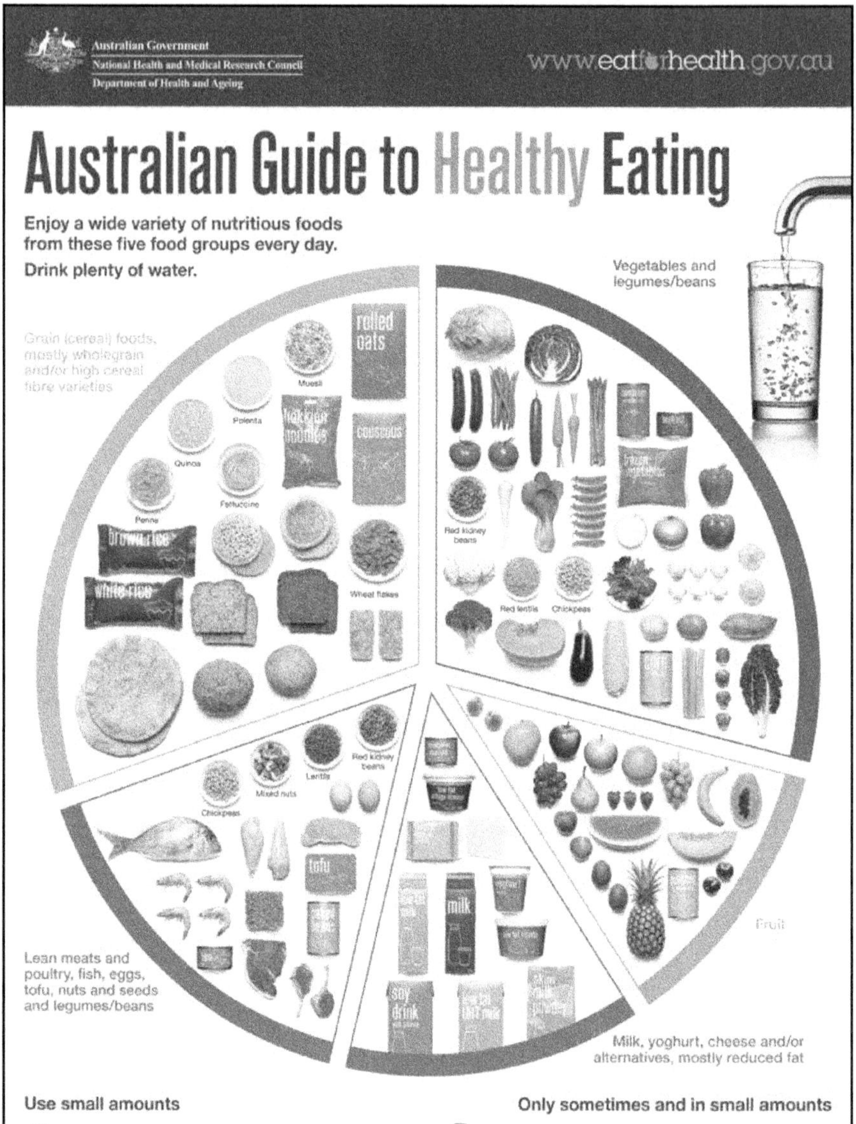

UNDERSTANDING FOOD LABELLING

Making informed decisions is imperative for good health. Food companies with their clever marketing will do anything and everything to get us to buy their products. Unfortunately, not everything you hear or see in an ad or read on the label these days is true. This is a problem, because misleading packaging and misinformation may be causing you to think you are making healthy food choices and decisions, however this may not be the case. And as a result, this could be affecting your weight, mood, energy levels, and sleep, and even worse, for those with children this misinformed eating can be passed down, creating a vicious cycle.

Does it really have fewer calories?

When a food item is labelled as 'fat free', 'low fat', or 'reduced fat', usually what that means is that without fat, the food would not taste good. And so, to make up for the low-fat taste, the food company adds in other ingredients such as sugar, salt, and thickeners, which add more calories. So, just because a food item says 'fat free' or 'low fat', that does not mean that it is necessarily healthy for you or has fewer calories. Sometimes it is even full of chemicals that you do not need.

Is it really organic?

Just because something is labelled 'organic' does not mean that it's necessarily organic or that it's good for you. This is where it pays dividends to do your research and make sure you are not just taking the word of the food companies, because they can be misleading. According to Australian Organic – the leading organic industry group in Australia – the term 'organic' is not currently regulated under Australian law. This means that companies are not required to follow specific regulations or an agreed standard to claim something is 'organic'. And as such, they caution consumers to always look for 'certified organic' products and a trusted certification logo, like their 'bud'.

Australian Organic also state that:

> To be certified organic means to grow or manufacture a product free from synthetic pesticides, herbicides, hormones and antibiotics. Livestock must be free to range and pasture-fed, seed must be non-GM, and the process must be water efficient and biodiversity friendly. Producers, processors, manufacturers and retailers of food, drink, fibre, skincare and cosmetics can be certified organic.

For answers to their FAQs, please follow this link: https://austorganic. com/about-us/faqs/.

FOOD IS NOT A REWARD OR A PUNISHMENT

Coming from Africa and growing up in the conditions that I did, it was very clear for me to see the vast difference between how children are brought up with food in Australia and the western world versus the part of Africa that I came from. I see what I describe as the vicious cycle. It is a cycle where children get rewarded with sugar, and unfortunately not knowing any better, those children then grow up and when they become parents themselves, they reward their own children with sugar also, and their children grow up and become parents and do the same thing, and on and on it goes. And this goes back generations. Those children that were given sweet treats or taken to the ice cream parlour or given lollies, biscuits, or chocolate as a reward for some good behaviour are parents and grandparents today. This was the way that they were shown love for doing something good, and now this is the same way they know how to treat their own children. This vicious cycle seems to be getting worse as the years go on, and it is something that needs to stop if we are serious about curbing the obesity rate in Australia and all the problems that come with making the wrong food choices.

Food is not a reward or a punishment. We should not give children junk food because they have behaved well or withhold it from them because they have not. Food is for the nourishment, sustenance, growth, and repair of our body. Junk food should only be treated as a 'sometimes' food, and the frequency should be kept to the very minimum otherwise it defeats the purpose.

PROTEIN SHAKES AND PRE-WORKOUT DRINKS

One question that I get asked all the time is, 'What protein shakes or pre-workout drinks do you have, Kay?' I believe the reason I get asked this question is firstly, because everyone nowadays is looking for some sort of 'secret', a 'shortcut' or way that they can get what they want in the quickest way possible with the least amount of effort. So, to look like I do, to many there must be some kind of magic drink that I take. Secondly, another reason why I get asked this question is because I probably look like one of the poster boys of the billion-dollar protein and pre-workout drinks industry. Every fitness magazine, fitness model, and bodybuilder seems to be promoting some sort of drink. This creates the impression they achieved their bodies with the help of those drinks, and their endorsement of those drinks alone make people think that if I want to look like him or her then I have to drink what he or she is drinking. And lastly, for some I believe it is purely out of curiosity. They may be thinking about starting their own exercise journey and are not sure where to begin, so they think or get told by someone that if they want to build muscles then they must take supplements.

A lot of people are surprised when I respond to their question that I do not drink any pre-workout drinks or protein shakes. I used to for a little while, but I quit drinking them and I will share my experience later on in this step. Everything we need to be successful in life is already within us. I passionately believe this.

Are they good for you?

Personally, I don't think so. I think they are full of sugar and chemicals that the body does not need. I understand 100% that not everyone will agree with my view on these drinks, since it seems like every gym-goer is drinking some sort of supplement these days. The pre-workout drinks are full of caffeine – you just have to see how many people drink coffee then you will understand why they are so popular. With sometimes quadruple the amount of caffeine compared to a standard cup of coffee, you get that instant feeling like it is working. Some pre-workout drinks are also full of chemicals – the likes that come up positive on drug tests. When I worked in the mines, there were workmates who tested positive during random drug tests when all they had taken was a pre-workout drink to give them energy. Some get you so high that they make your body all jittery, and when they wear off they leave you feeling very flat.

The protein shakes are full of sugar, which I sort of get the idea of. After your workout, when you have depleted all your energy stores, you need fast-releasing sugar to replenish your blood sugar level – but how much of this is too much? You have people drinking multiple protein shakes a day. One drink is not enough anymore. Some gym-goers have pre-workout, intra-workout, and post-workout shakes. Seriously, how much can your body handle? What happened to real food?

If you must have some sort of drink to make you feel like you are doing something, I recommend you look for organic, healthier alternatives and not the ones that are full of chemicals. Most times if you cannot pronounce the name of the ingredient, that is a clear sign that you should stay clear.

Are they worth the money?

To be honest with you, I think they are a waste of money. Unless of course you're medically required to have dietary supplements. Anyone who takes pre-workout drinks and protein shakes will tell you that they are not cheap. And this was one of the reasons

I questioned taking those drinks. When I realised how much they were costing me, I had to stop and think, and I realised that I did not really need them. I have seen weightlifters who have not had a single pre-workout or protein shake in their life and they were able to build huge muscles, even bigger than the majority of gym-goers who drink pre-workout drinks and protein shakes.

Before moving to Australia, I worked out with guys back in Africa in our makeshift gym and these guys were huge. We did not even know what a pre-workout drink was, or a protein shake.

MY OWN EXPERIMENT WITH SUPPLEMENTS

When I first moved here to Australia and started going to the gym, taking supplements seemed like a thing that everyone did. It was a norm. All the gyms had buckets of powders – pre-workout, intra-workout, and post-workout drinks. So, I felt like I needed to take them too. At first, I could not afford to buy them, so I just trained. But as soon as I could afford it, I bought my first bucket of protein powder and then some pre-workout powders also. At some stage I was even taking some intra-workout creatine. I even pro-moted these supplements. (I chuckle at myself just thinking about that.) So, for about three years, I took supplements.

In 2012, I began to question taking these supplements. This was around the time that supplements containing DMAA (dimeth-ylamylamine) were being banned across the US and Canada due to links to deaths from heart attack. So, I decided to do some research. According to the University of Colorado, adequate protein supple-mentation is not necessary if you have access to a diet that is healthy and contains adequate nutrients. The research also suggested that pre-workout drinks can cause liver damage, diarrhoea, kidney dam-age, and cardiac arrest. This is due to the high dosage of caffeine, creatine and other ingredients, which can cause stress on your heart.

I knew how pre-workouts made me feel. They boosted my energy level – I mean, with the amount of caffeine present in a pre-workout drink it was no surprise. I also did not like how flat they made me feel after they had worn off. And I did not like how much they were costing me.

So, I started to do some experiments with myself. The first one I did was to prove to myself whether or not I really needed these supplements. What I did was to completely go off all supplements and try to redo all the heaviest lifts I had ever done to that point. It turned out that I lifted even heavier weights while I was not taking any supplements. I have gained more muscles since I stopped taking supplements.

When I stopped taking supplements in 2012, I weighed 85 kilograms. In 2014 I got up to 94 kilograms of body weight, and that is the heaviest I have weighed, and I can tell you that it was not fat. I now weigh between 92 and 94 kilos. I could train to get heavier, but I like staying around 90 kilos. It means that I can do things that are important to me like being able to get up tomorrow and run 5 or 10 kilometres without suffering too much, or train for a half or full marathon and jump up 60 or more inches high.

'KAY, WHAT CAN I DO TO LOSE MY BEER BELLY?'

This is a question I get asked a lot, and it sometimes comes in different forms. It does not always end with 'beer belly'. Most times it is like, 'Kay, what exercises can I do to lose my stomach?'

Back in 2012 when I first started Muscle Garden Personal Training, a friend of mine asked me, 'Kay, mate what can I do to lose my beer belly?' I simply answered his question with another question. I responded: 'Have you ever considered losing the beer first?' You see, sometimes the solution we seek lies within the problem. If you have a belly because you think you are drinking too much beer, the logical thing to do, if you really want to reduce your belly, is to reduce the amount of beer you drink, or cut it out altogether. Sometimes we look for quick fixes to solve a problem because we do not want to face the hard facts. We do not want to do the things that will take us outside of our comfort zones. But outside of our comfort zones is where the results are. Weight loss, muscle gain, more energy, good health, being a good role model, achieving the body that you can be happy with. All of these things come with some form of sacrifice. You have to give something of yourself to get what you want. You have to make changes and you have to prioritise the things that are more important for your health and for your quality of life. Nothing worth having in life comes easy. If it was easy, it would not be worth it. Changing your diet and limiting or cutting out foods you have eaten your whole life will be one of the hardest things you will ever do, so you have to ask yourself: what is the reward? Is it worth it? How is it going to change my life for the better? What impact is it going to have on the people around me? 'How Bad Do You Want It?'

Getting noticeably clear on these questions will help you stay the course. If you are determined enough, you will achieve your goal. And being determined does not mean you will not have bad days or shortfalls; it means that regardless of your shortfalls, you can still pick yourself up and keep going.

FOOD AND GROWING UP IN AFRICA

Africa is one of the poorest continents in the world. And when you think about Africa, generally what comes to mind is poverty, sicknesses and diseases, civil wars, and something a little positive – the safaris and natural resources. I grew up in West Africa, and though the living conditions were tough compared to the western world, there are some good things that I liked about growing up in Africa:

- **Food came from the earth and the field.** We ate food that came from the ground, the fields, from the rivers or oceans. We did not have pesticides sprayed on nearly everything we ate. The meat was not made to last with chemicals – it was either smoked or salted – and food did not travel in trucks from thousands of miles away. If you wanted to cook greens or chicken, you just had to go in the garden near the house or grab one of your own chickens running around. And if you did not have these, you just had to go to the markets where the majority of the food sold came from people's own farms and gardens.

- **No McDonald's or fast-food TV ads.** One of the things I now love about growing up in the parts of Africa that I did is that TV screens were not littered with junk food ads. Kids were not brainwashed right from a young age to consume junk food. In regional towns like Mackay and Townsville, sporting teams and sporting events are sponsored by McDonald's; Sponsorship is a good thing, but it is a way to constantly keep their products and brand in your face.

PREPARATION – A KEY INGREDIENT

A busy schedule is one of the most common reasons that people use when admitting to not making time to exercise. It is also one of the most common reasons why people opt for takeaway or drive-through meals on their way home from work.

Amidst busy schedules, competing priorities and tight budgets, being prepared is one of the most effective tools to stay on track, within budget and make progress towards your goals. Meal and exercise planning are a sure way to achieve this.

Meal planning involves taking the time to decide on the meals you will eat over the course of the week and putting them into a weekly meal plan template. From this template, you can reflect on your meal choices and make changes where necessary. I love meal planning because it keeps you organised, helps you minimise unnecessary splurges on take out, and it helps you save money on your grocery shop. Following is an easy guide for you to follow that will help you plan your meals in advance, as well as help you make good decisions and think about what you eat.

muscle garden
health & fitness centre

"A gym for everyday people"

Notes

Meal Options

Breakfast – 6am

1.
2.
3.
4.
5.

Morning Snack – 9am

1.
2.
3.
4.
5.

Lunch – 12pm

1.
2.
3.
4.
5.

Afternoon Snack – 3pm

1.
2.
3.
4.
5.

Dinner – 6pm

1.
2.
3.
4.
5.

Evening Snack (optional)

1.
2.
3.
4.
5.

Note: Time doesn't have to be exact. If you can work within the 3hr range that will be great!

Weekly Meal Planner Template

muscle garden
health & fitness centre
"A gym for everyday people"

Week No: ___ Date Range: ___	Monday	Tuesday	Wednesday	Thursday	Friday	Saturday	Sunday
Breakfast 6am							
Morning Snack 9am							
Lunch 12pm							
Afternoon Snack 3pm							
Dinner 6pm							
Evening Snack 9pm							

Note: The time is just an indication and doesn't have to be exact. If you can keep your meals within the 3hr range that will help you achieve your goals.

MY FAMILY RECIPES

'What do you eat, Kay?'

People often ask me this question because I believe they attribute my physique to what I eat. This is partly true, but I like to think that I look the way I do because of what I do *not* eat or drink. Like, for example, I do not drink alcohol. That is something that most people would struggle to give up. Though I do not preach that people should quit drinking, reducing your alcohol consumption can make a difference to your waistline. I do not eat junk food. But I do eat rice, bread, fruit and vegetables, poultry, beef, and salads, but my guess is that is not what you want to know. So, to help you to get started on your own journey of healthy eating (and to appease your curiosity), I have included in appendix A some of our family recipes from my wife's upcoming recipe book titled *Our Family Eats*. It is our hope that these will not only give you an idea of what I eat but will also help you with your diet. We hope you find them useful.

STEP 4

GET LOTS OF
EXERCISE
TO LIVE A LIFE FULL OF
ENERGY AND VITALITY

YOUR GARDEN OF MUSCLES

The name Muscle Garden is drawn from the analogy between a garden of plants and the human body. I believe the human body is a garden of muscles. We have over 640 different muscles in our body, grouped into cardiac muscles (muscles of your heart), skeletal muscles (muscles of your arms, legs, back and so on), and smooth muscles (muscles lining the walls of your blood vessels). And just as we would look after our garden of plants by watering it, fertilising it, exposing it to sunlight, getting rich soil for it, plucking the weeds, and pruning it if we wanted our garden of plants to bloom, flourish, and look admirable, so too with our body – our garden of muscles.

If we want to look and feel great and help to ward off diseases such as obesity, diabetes, osteoporosis, depression and anxiety, and certain types of cancers, we have to look after our garden of muscles with proper nutrition and exercise. This will in turn give us the energy we need to run around with our children or grandchildren, the strength we need to get through our daily activities, the mental clarity to think quickly, and the self-esteem we need to live our best lives.

Muscle Garden is the name of my business, but it is not a building with four walls. Muscle Garden is *you*. Your body is a garden of muscles, and it is my hope that you begin to look at yourself this way. How you treat your garden will determine the results you get.

THE IMPORTANCE OF EXERCISE

Exercise is especially important because your quality of life depends on it.

When we exercise on a regular basis, we improve our blood pressure, we sleep better, and we have more energy and vitality. We can run around with our children or grandchildren, we improve our self-esteem, we are better equipped to fight diseases and we get to live longer. We lose weight when we exercise, we build muscles, and we get stronger, fitter, and live a happy, healthy life.

Exercise is defined as any bodily activity that enhances and maintains physical fitness and wellness. Whether it is walking, running, swimming, lifting weights, or playing sport, at some stage in your life you have probably done some form of exercise, if not currently.

Exercise is performed for various reasons, including:

- improving cardiovascular health
- weight loss or maintaining a healthy weight
- muscle growth
- developing strong bones and muscles
- reducing ageing
- enhancing athletic skills
- improving mood and mental clarity.

Our body was made to move.

THE MANY BENEFITS OF EXERCISE

It improves your physical appearance

I have been in business for over eight years now and the life-changing power of exercise that I have seen with my clients blows me away every time. I have helped hundreds of clients lose weight over the years, and to see a client completely transform into someone who looks like a totally different person altogether is amazing. It does not matter how many times I have seen these transformations; the amazement is always new because each client is different with their own set of challenges.

Overcoming those challenges to achieve a goal that they did not think was possible before gives me chills every time. Take Stephen and Chantel, for example. Stephen lost 56 kilos and became completely unrecognisable from the person he used to be. Chantel lost

31 kilos and same thing: she looked like a different person. Their physical appearance improved dramatically. They gained muscles which made them stronger; you began to see muscle definition which was not apparent before. They developed strong bones and muscles, which enabled them to carry out their daily tasks more efficiently, and their posture was significantly better. They could stand tall and upright.

It boosts your energy levels and vitality

When I think about exercising or lifting weights, I cannot pinpoint exactly why I started. Other than the fact that I loved the feeling, it was something else to do to fill my time. Unlike most people, and contrary to what I now preach, I never went to the gym with a goal. And that will explain why I cannot tell you exactly why I started training. I simply fell in love with working out. I loved the feeling of exercising. Especially the feeling of hypertrophy – the increase in size of muscle cells as a result of the blood flow to that particular muscle you are training with weights – commonly known as 'the pump'. For me, back then it did not matter whether I built muscles or not, lose weight or not. I just had to turn up and train. In doing so, I built muscles, I got stronger, I got fitter.

Today, if you were to ask me why I exercise, the answer is truly clear as day. Having an abundance of energy and vitality to run my business and still being able to be an engaging husband and father is of paramount concern to me. Exercise does that for me. It gives me the energy I need to be both productive at work and at home. And this is something I have seen with my clients as well.

When Wayne first came to see me in 2015 for personal training, his main goal was to improve his energy levels during the day and sleep better at night. He believed achieving this goal would help him become more productive at work. And he was not wrong. Wayne is an accountant, and he runs his own business as well as having a beautiful family of four. I am no accountant, but I can imagine it would be a stressful job.

Since 2015 to the writing of this book, Wayne has been a client of mine. To say that he never gets tired or does not have a bad night's sleep here and there would be far from the truth, but for the majority of the time Wayne is now full of energy and vitality. He gets a good night's rest and is at the top his game, delivering remarkable results for his clients as well as for his business and family.

And when Steve lost 56 kilos of body fat, he noticed that instead of struggling to barely get through a 12-hour shift at work, he was now working up to 16 hours a day with plenty of energy to spare. That is the wonder of exercise.

It helps you set a good example for your children or loved ones to follow

My son Malachi was barely a year old when he started copying me doing exercises. I still remember the first day he started to do push-ups. Then he went on to start doing burpees and jumping on the machines at the gym and copying what he saw. As he grew a little older, he started joining me in the backyard to do some of my back-yard workouts.

When children are little they learn through imitation and mod-elling, or what is known as 'observational learning'. And parents are their number one teacher. While it is true that children may not always copy exactly what they see, they will copy the behaviours that are rewarded or done repeatedly. This is why it is particularly important to set good examples for children to follow, especially from an early age. My son Malachi may grow up one day and decide exercise is not his thing, but while he is young and has an interest in doing exercises, it's my responsibility to keep rewarding him every time he does so. Sometimes I jokingly tell him that he will be the fastest man in the world one day and that he will 'carve people up'. Every now and then, he will come over and say, 'Daddy, see how fast I can run', then he will sprint off.

Research shows that children with healthy parents are 75% more likely to end up living a healthy lifestyle. The fact that both his mother and I exercise, and him being surrounded by exercise and growing up in a gym, makes it easy for him.

The flow-on effect of exercise does not just stop with children; it has an impact on adults as well. I have seen clients whose relatives decided to take up exercise and change their lives just from seeing the results that their husbands, wives, adult children, parents, or friends were able to achieve. I run a fitness facility that is family focused, and I see this all the time.

It improves your self-esteem and confidence

For the most part of 2014 and 2015 I trained a client named Justin. He had a friendly and jovial personality, and just from looking at Justin, you would not think that he was self-conscious.

Justin would always wear long track pants to training. I never bothered to ask why. In fact, it did not matter as long as they did not restrict him from doing his exercise activities. It was not a big deal, until one day Justin came to training wearing shorts – something I had never seen him do before. Justin had been taking notice of his improvements. He noticed that his leg muscles had grown in size and that he could now see his muscle definition. He wore shorts purposely that day to show me his muscles. He was proud of his achievement, and so was I. He allowed me to take photos of his leg muscle definition and post them on our business's Facebook page to serve as an inspiration to others. He felt confident enough to show his legs and did not feel the need to cover them up anymore. From that day, I did not see him wear his usual long track pants to training.

Lucy was another example. She was a client of mine who only wore T-shirts to training every day and covered up as much as she could. She did not feel confident enough to wear singlets. I remember when she partook in her first Mackay Marina Run as part of Team Muscle Garden; we only had singlets made that year. She wore a T-shirt under her singlet. But after she had lost weight and started to see muscle definition in her arms, I saw her wear a singlet to training for the first time without a T-shirt under it.

I have also seen a lot of clients go from being self-conscious about their ability to do certain exercises or even about joining a group training session to being very confident as a result of stepping outside of their comfort zones and achieving results they did not think possible. Even clients who did not feel confident going for social runs or bike rides with colleagues or friends would now do so.

One of the things I have found that helps me and many of my clients improve self-esteem and confidence is improving physical appearance, and exercise is a great way to do that.

It helps you live a better quality of life

Exercise, or the lack of, can be the determining factor in whether we have the energy and fitness to run around with our children, how we perform at work, how we carry out our day-to-day activities, how we move about, how we sleep, and whether or not in our senior years we use a cane, a walker, a motorised chair, or move about freely.

Exercise does not only help to strengthen our muscles, it also helps to strengthen our bones, it improves our joints, our mood, our flexibility and mobility; it helps us to lose weight, to be fitter, stronger and faster, and all of these things help us to enjoy life to the fullest.

When Stephen came to see me, he weighed over 140 kilos. The doctor had told him that if he wanted to be around longer to play with his grandchildren, he needed to do something about his health. Stephen did not move as freely as he did when he got down to 86 kilos. He could now work longer hours and be more productive. He could now go on holidays with his wife and ride through the desert in the middle of Australia with relative ease compared to what he had been able to do before.

Take Wayne for another example. A painter by trade, Wayne confessed that he always had lower back pain. Lower back pain is one of the most annoying pains you can experience. It is so prevalent among people today that estimates from the Australian Bureau of Statistics 2017–18 National Health Survey showed that about

4 million Australians (16% of the population) have back problems. It's estimated that 70% to 90% of people will suffer from lower back pain in some form at some point in their lives. Through exercise, Wayne was able to strengthen his back and was able to do his job easily, as well enjoy life without having to worry about being sore all the time.

It helps you prevent or manage depression and anxiety

Published in 2017 in the *American Journal of Psychiatry*, the Black Dog Institute led a study which found that 12% of cases of depression could have been prevented by doing one hour of physical activity per week. The landmark study revealed that regular exercise of any intensity can prevent future depression. The study was the largest and most extensive of its kind; it involved 33,908 Norwegian adults who had their levels of exercise and symptoms of depression and anxiety monitored over 11 years.

Depression is a constant feeling of sadness and loss of interest in doing your normal activities. There are different types of depression with varying degrees of symptoms, from minor to severe. Depression is common. In any one-year period, around one million people in Australia experience depression. One in six women and one in eight men will experience depression at some point in their life.

At the writing of this book, according to data from the Beyond Blue website:

3 million Australians are living with depression or anxiety. Anxiety is the most common mental health condition in Australia, and on average, one in four people – one in three women and one in five men – will experience anxiety at some stage in their life. In a 12-month period, over 2 million Australians experience anxiety.

One of the known ways to help manage anxiety and depression is living a healthy lifestyle that involves keeping active.

I have had clients who came to see me for training not because they wanted to lose weight, not because they wanted to build muscle or get fit, but simply because they wanted to manage their mental health. They understood the importance of exercise and the role it played in helping them stay in top mental capacity. To them, losing weight or building muscle or getting fit was a by-product of their actions, and whether or not that happened, it was not their concern. Their concern was their mental health.

It helps to improve your quality of sleep

The number of times I have heard people say, 'I slept like a baby' the day after they have done a workout is countless. In my research for this topic, I found there is a substantial body of evidence that exercise helps improve sleep. Dr Shawn D. Youngstedt, PHD of the University of South Carolina, in his research paper published in 2005, states: 'Historically, perhaps no daytime behaviour has been more closely associated with better sleep than exercise.' And one of the reasons why exercise is so important when it comes to helping us sleep better is because no other stimulus creates a greater depletion of energy stores, tissue breakdown, and elevation of body temperature. Sleep helps us to replenish all of these things. It helps us conserve energy, restore broken-down tissues, and down-regulate our body temperature.

According to many research papers, regular exercise helps to improve your sleep quality – you have deep, restful sleeps. It also helps you sleep longer – it prolongs the amount of time you spend sleeping. And it can help with sleep disorders like insomnia. And all you need is as little as 30 minutes of exercise per day or a total of 150 minutes spread out through the week.

What I have found over my years of exercising is that, even though I wake up early every day, I mostly have a good night's sleep, and that is very important to me because it helps me function properly. For someone who does not drink coffee, I need all the energy

I can get to last through the day of being a husband, father, business owner, employer, and a servant to my community. And I get that from exercise and a good night's sleep.

It helps you prevent or manage diseases

When Kel came to see me for personal training in 2015, he had already had three stents inserted into his heart to prevent him from having a heart attack. A stent is a tiny tube inserted into a blocked passageway to keep it open so that the flow of blood and fluids are restored. In addition to that, Kel's lung capacity was also restricted to 42%.

Prior to Kel coming to see me, his wife Leone was already a client of mine. Leone suffers scoliosis and was experiencing constant back pain. Leone found that exercise helped her cope with the pain and gave her the strength to do her daily activities. Seeing her results with regular exercise, she believed that it would be good for her husband Kel. She arranged a consultation for Kel and he immediately began training.

At first Kel could not do a lot. We had to gradually work him into exercising to help him get through a session. We would have frequent breaks so that Kel could catch his breath.

Through regular training, along with his medication, Kel was able to increase his lung capacity up to 85%. His doctor told him that whatever he was doing was working and that he should keep it up. His strength level was dramatically improved. Kel went from not being able to squat a 20-kilo bar to squatting 100 kilos and deadlifting 120 kilos. But these numbers meant nothing more than the fact that Kel was now living a very fit and healthy lifestyle. He could lift things at work that he had previously struggled to lift. He could do simple things without quickly running out of breath. Kel was able to manage his condition quite well by exercising on a regular basis.

YOUR HEALTH IS AN INVESTMENT NOT AN EXPENSE

I sit down with people almost on a daily basis to discuss their health goals and why it is important for them to start exercising, and often I find out that by not exercising, it is *costing* them something. Something especially important to them, and that something is not money. Sometimes it is lack of self-esteem due to being overweight, and other times it's a lack of better sleep – they struggle to have restful sleep, resulting in low energy, not being able to be productive at work or play with their children, and the list goes on. I often tell them that the actual cost is where they are right now versus where they want to get to. And then I tell them there is a price to pay. Again, that price is not money. For personal training clients, that price is they have to come see me or one of our trainers at least three times a week for training, and sometimes they are not going to like feeling sore or out of breath due to training, but that is the price they have to pay. That is what they have to do to get to where they want to get to. Discomfort precedes success. And then there is an investment that they have to make for their health, and that is paying us to use our expertise to help them achieve that better quality of life, or whatever their goal may be.

Think about this. What is your inactivity costing you?

If you have the motivation to exercise on your own, find a fitness facility that is supportive and welcoming and that is willing to write a program for you to help you with your health and fitness goals.

If you do not trust yourself with motivation then my advice will be to get a personal trainer who knows what they are doing and who can help you achieve your goals, and make the commitment to invest in your health.

If fitness facilities and personal trainers are not your thing, then buy a pair of runners and go for a walk, jog, or run. Take up swimming or cycling. Anything. It doesn't matter what you do, as long as you do *something*.

Remember your health is an investment *not* an expense.

How Bad Do You Want It?

'I WANT TO LOSE WEIGHT: SHOULD I DO CARDIO OR LIFT WEIGHTS?'

As a personal trainer and gym owner, this is another question I get asked a lot, and rightfully so. There are people – including trainers – who are pro cardio and some who are pro weights. But I, on the other hand, recommend doing both. And there is a good reason why. There is no doubt that any exercise is good for you. And these two types of exercise are certainly great for losing weight. They both have their advantages and disadvantages when it comes to their effect on weight loss.

Let's take an example: I weigh over 90 kilograms at the writing of this step. The last time I went for a five-kilometre run, I burned 554 calories in 21 minutes and 41 seconds with an average heart rate of 167 beats per minute. Someone heavier than me may burn more than that number of calories within that time. Now, if I were to strength train for that same amount of time, there is no way I would have burned 554 calories within 21 minutes. Per minute, cardio burns more calories. So, in this case, if we were to base the effectiveness of weight loss purely on the number of calories burned during the session, cardio would have the leg up. Another advantage of cardiovascular exercises like running, cycling, or swimming is that you get to keep your heart rate up over a sustained period of time, much more than what you would do if you were doing weights.

With that being said, though you may not burn more calories during the session as cardio, strength training keeps your metabolism elevated long after your workout, which helps you burn more calories. Strength training also helps you build muscle mass. For every 2.3 kilos of muscle you gain, you can burn up to 250 calories at rest.

I recommend doing both because that's how you get the most benefit. You get to lose fat as well as improve your shape. If you just want to lose fat, cardio is great as you burn more calories per session, but if you want to lose fat as well as build muscles and improve your physical appearance and be functionally fit and strong, then do both.

Researchers at Duke University conducted the largest study of its kind to find an answer to which was most effective for weight loss. After eight months of tracking 119 overweight and previously sedentary volunteers while they did strength training, cardio, or a combination of both, those who did just cardio lost more weight than those who did just strength training. Though they spent more time in the gym, those who did both strength training and cardio had the most improved body composition. They lost the most body fat and added more lean muscle mass to their body.

WHAT ARE YOUR EXERCISE OPTIONS?

Weight training

Weight training can interchangeably be referred to as strength training, weightlifting, or resistance training.

I know that sometimes when people think of weightlifting, they think of big, bulging muscles. I hear this all the time: 'I do not want to lift weights because I do not want to build big muscles.' That is far from the truth. You are not going to build big muscles overnight from lifting weights. If you are not already doing so, I encourage you to lift weights because weight, strength, or resistance training is especially important. Unlike some cardiovascular exercises, weight training helps us to preserve muscle mass. Due to sarcopenia (loss of muscle with ageing) we lose up to about 5% of our muscle mass each decade after the age of 20. Ageing is inevitable, and so is muscle loss that comes with ageing, but we can slow down this process by lifting weights.

Weightlifting also helps with weight loss. When we lift weights, we help to improve our metabolism, and an improved metabolism helps us to burn more calories because the body works harder to maintain muscles than it does with fat.

Strength training helps to prevent or manage osteoporosis (a condition causing weak and fragile bones). By doing strength training on a regular basis we help to increase our bone density, and this helps us build stronger bones which then leads us to avoiding or managing osteoporosis.

Resistance training helps to decrease our risk of injuries. When we train with resistance, we strengthen our muscles and protect our joints, and this helps us to minimise our risk of injuries.

Weightlifting is more than just big biceps and a squat-booty, so I hope you include some weightlifting into your exercise routine if you are not already doing so.

Cardiovascular exercise

Cardio – as it is known – or aerobic exercise is physical exercise ranging from low to high intensity that is based solely on the use of the aerobic energy system. Aerobic means relating to, involving, or requiring free oxygen. When we perform aerobic exercises such as walking, jogging, running, swimming, cycling, or rowing at a low to moderate intensity, our heart pumps oxygenated blood to our muscles to meet the demand. Aerobic exercises are generally designed to be performed at light to moderate intensities for an extended period of time, to avoid the build up of lactic acid, and so that all carbohydrates are aerobically turned into energy. This usually builds aerobic endurance.

Cardio exercises primarily or exclusively involve the use of the legs. Using the rowing machine, a cross trainer, an air-bike, a skipping rope, boxing, and battle ropes – for example – involve other muscles like the arms, back, shoulders, chest, and abdominals.

Aerobic exercise is commonly mixed up with *anaerobic* exercise. Common examples of *anaerobic* exercise are strength training and short distance running or sprinting, as I would prefer to call it. The two types of exercise are different in terms of duration, how energy is generated within the muscles, and the intensity of the muscle contraction.

Some of the benefits of doing cardiovascular or aerobic exercise are:

- strengthening and enlarging the muscles of the heart
- strengthening the muscles involved in breathing to help with the flow of oxygen in and out of the lungs
- improving circulation
- increasing the number of red blood cells, making it easy for the body to transport oxygen from the lungs into the blood and muscles.

It also helps with reducing the risk of diabetes and other diseases.

Calisthenics

'Calisthenics' comes from the ancient Greek words 'kalos' – meaning 'beauty' or 'beautiful' – and 'sthenos' – meaning 'strength'. Combined, they mean beautiful strength, which is the art of using one's own body weight as resistance to build strength and physique. Examples of calisthenic exercise include:

- push-ups
- pull-ups or chin-ups
- body weight squats
- sit-ups
- burpees
- dips
- handstands
- planks
- shuttle runs
- muscle-ups
- leg raises.

Calisthenics helps to not only build strength and physique, but it also helps to build aerobic capacity, flexibility, balance, agility, and coordination.

What I love about calisthenics is that it requires minimal to no equipment to get a workout done. Even though I own two gyms and do understand the importance of the gym, I do not believe it is the only means by which you can get fit. I often post on my social media pages a variety of body weight exercise routines that I perform in my backyard or outdoors because I want my followers to be inspired to look at their backyard or exercise in general in a different way.

There are a ton of exercises that can be done without you having to set foot in a gym. Sometimes it's as simple as starting with a little shuttle jog in your backyard for warmup, then following that up with some push-ups, body weight squats and then sit-ups. You could even throw in some burpees if you want to challenge yourself a little bit more. You can pick, say, 5 to 10 repetitions and then do that for about 3 to 5 sets depending on your level of fitness.

The health benefits of exercising far outweigh the risks of not exercising. And calisthenic exercises provide the means for people to exercise without having to buy a gym membership or expensive home gym equipment which they may not use long term due to lack of motivation. However, the social aspect of training in a gym and meeting new friends and likeminded people can create stickiness to your exercise journey.

Plyometrics

Have you ever seen someone jump over a box before, or jump from a box down onto the ground and then explode straight back up? That's plyometrics. It can also be referred to as 'jump training'. Plyometrics are exercises that put your muscles under maximum force or effort within short periods of time to help build speed and strength or power. Originally meant for athletes, sprinters, and high jumpers, the term is now very common within the fitness world.

Fred Wilt, a former US Olympic long-distance runner, was the American who came up with the name 'plyometrics'. After watching the Russians do jumps in their warmups, he wondered why they were doing all these jumps while they – the Americans – were only doing static stretches. He believed the jumps were responsible for their success.

Plyometrics is one form of training that I very much use in my own training regime, as well as with clients. It is explosive, quick, and it puts your muscles under extreme force to perform. One of my claims to fame in Mackay and surroundings is my TV ad where I jump over wheelie bins. Everywhere I go, there is usually someone who will come up to me and ask: 'Are you that guy who jumps over wheelie bins on TV?'

So how did the wheelie bin ad come about? In 2012, part of my training heavily involved plyometrics. I had multiple boxes built for doing box jumps. Sometimes I would do more than 200 box jumps in one session. I would then line up five or more boxes and jump onto and over them, performing certain numbers of repetitions at a time. And other times, I would stack the boxes on top of each other and jump onto them, jump down, and then explode straight back up again atop the boxes. I would stack a 24-inch box onto a 20-inch box and jump onto or over them. I never considered stacking a 24-inch box onto another 24-inch box and jumping onto them until one day a client asked me if I could.

Instead of answering with words, I wanted show him, and prove to myself whether I could or not. To be honest, even I was not sure if I could pull it off, so it was going to be great finding out. I stacked the boxes and attempted the jump. As it turned I had enough explosive power in my legs to get on top of 48 inches. That became my new personal best, and a new standard for box jumps was born.

During this time, I worked out of a friend's gym which was tied to their church as well as a charity organisation. They had a lot of wheelie bins to cater for the church, charity, as well as the gym. I would see all the bins lined up on bin day, and one day the thought crossed my mind: *what would it feel like to line up at least five bins in a row and jump over them one at a time?* So that is exactly what I did.

One afternoon, I lined up five bins in a row and asked my mate to film me jumping over them. I put the video on my social media page, and it caught a lot of buzz. But it was not until 2015 that I decided to make it into a TV ad. I thought there was nothing like it on TV, and that it was something everyone would be able to relate to considering every home had a bin. I had no idea the ad would be as successful as it was.

I have since gone on to jump way higher than 48 inches. My point is, had it not been for me including plyometrics or jump training into my routines I would not have had the strength and speed to perform those jumps.

High Intensity Interval Training

High Intensity Interval Training, or HIIT for short, is a form of interval training where one or more exercises are performed with an all-out effort for a period ranging from 20 to 90 seconds or more, interspersed with short recovery times. Depending on the program, the duration may last for about 30 to 45 minutes, depending on the fitness level of participants.

HIIT sessions help to improve overall strength and condition as well as reduce body fat mass. The types of exercises performed in a HIIT session vary. A typical HIIT session may involve a bike, treadmill or track, a sled, boxing with a bag or partner, cross trainer, and battle ropes.

HIIT sessions can also be in the form of circuit training, where you have a number of exercises in a circuit. You perform one exercise for time, have a little break, then move on to the next exercise until the whole circuit is complete.

There are different types of HIIT training. The most common one today is the Tabata training based on a 1996 study done by Professor Izumi Tabata. Tabata training involves doing an exercise at high intensity for 20 seconds, then having 10 seconds break, then doing it again and again continuously for eight rounds – a total of four minutes. This form of HIIT gave birth to other forms of interval training that may follow the pattern of 30 seconds on and 30 seconds off for a number of rounds, or 45 seconds on and 15 seconds off, and so on.

Though HIIT sessions predominantly involve the use of cardiovascular exercises, the same principle can be applied to other forms of training. Say, for example, I can do barbell back squats for 20 seconds and have a 10-second break, and do that several times, or do a bench press for as many reps as I can within 30 seconds then have a 30-second break and then go again for a number of rounds. I might decide to do box jumps for 30 seconds on and 30 seconds off.

You get the idea – the principle of high intensity training can be applied to other forms of training as well as different exercises.

'I HAVE NEVER SET FOOT IN A GYM BEFORE; HOW DO I GET STARTED?'

Get help

You have not got enough years in your life to learn from your own mistakes. If you have never been to a gym before, the experience can be quite daunting, especially if it is a mainstream gym. So, the best thing to do is to get some help. For example: as a business owner, I do not try to do my own tax, I have an accountant who does it for me. I do not try to service my own car, and I do not pretend to be a doctor when I am unwell. You get the point. That is the same thing with exercise. If you do not know what to do to help you get the results you want, find someone who knows and understands how to help you get there more quickly than you would on your own.

Find the right gym

There are so many gyms around today that offer different training needs for different people. The first thing you want to do before you join any gym is to find one that is the right fit for you, one that aligns with your values and, more importantly, one that offers what you are looking for in terms of training style.

Some people care about going to a gym where they feel part of something more than just a gym – like a family – somewhere they are treated like human beings and not just another number, while others do not. There are gyms that offer just group training – if this is something you are looking for, then good for you, but not everyone wants or feels comfortable in a group-training environment so this may not be the right fit for them. There are also gyms that offer both group training options as well a gym floor where you can go and do your own thing.

There are so many options to choose from these days with varying price points. If possible, do a free trial before you join, or do some research to find out more about the gym you are thinking about joining. See if they are what you want before you join. If you do not do this, you run a risk of joining a gym and not going.

Do a health screen

After joining a gym, you want to do a health screen to see where you are really starting from. If you really want to go deeper into knowing your body, it might be beneficial to get some blood tests done at your GP to find out where you are starting from, what your health status is, and what the areas are that you need to improve.

You can also ask your gym if they have a body composition analyser. This machine will help you understand not only your weight but how much of that weight is muscle and how much of it is fat, as well as tell you how they are distributed around your body. It will tell you how much water you carry in your body in litres, how much skeletal muscle mass (muscles on your bones) and body fat mass you have, and many other important details that you will need to know before you get started. The reason for this is that generally you cannot manage what you cannot measure. This information will arm you with what you need to do to improve your results or see how you are tracking. You'll see whether you are progressing or not, and if not, what you can do to improve. And importantly, it helps you understand what truly lies beneath the surface, as the scales do not usually tell you the full story.

Get some personal training

Most people after joining the gym for the first time or after a long break decide to get some personal training sessions to give them a kickstart and the push they need to help them form a new habit. The personal trainer helps point them in the right direction, arming them with tools and information they will need to carry on by themselves.

Others prefer to not have to worry about having to do it themselves. So, they hire a personal trainer to help them achieve their goals. I have clients who have been doing personal training with me for five-plus years and counting. For them it is the accountability that matters – if they have a session booked, they are likely to show up at the gym, but if they do not, they probably will not. It's also the peace of mind knowing that they do not have to worry about doing it by themselves. They can just show up, get trained by an expert, and then leave.

While personal training may not be something that everyone can afford, it is a great way to fast track your results. It is an investment in yourself that is worth making. Personal training nowadays can be done either face to face or online. With the online version, you will be assigned training programs along with videos to explain the exercises. After you have completed the exercises, you tick 'complete' to let your trainer know that you have done the exercise, as a means of accountability.

As with everything, remember not all personal trainers are worth their weight in gold. Find one who knows and understands what they are doing and is experienced in helping their clients achieve the results they are after.

Get a program

If you have never been to a gym before then after joining you will want to have a detailed gym program created for you to help you achieve your goals. Most gyms will give a one-page program with about five exercises and expect that program to help you achieve your goals. The reality of what happens is that, after a couple of weeks, you get bored with that piece of paper and your motivation drops.

Find a gym that will spend the time needed with you to put together a program that aligns with your goals. Some gyms will offer this for free, but even if you must pay for it that's fine; this will help guide you on the right path and give you the peace of mind of knowing that when you walk into the gym you have a plan to follow, which is something to look forward to. Make sure to have it updated periodically and track your progress along the way.

The most important thing to remember about getting a program done is that it should help you get to your goal. If your goal is to be fit so you can run five kilometres in less than 25 minutes by a certain date, your program should cater for that. If your goal is to be strong so that you can deadlift 100 kilograms by a certain date, then your program should cater for that. Whatever your goal is, your program should be aligned to suit. Your goal might be that you are a busy person and you have limited time to spend in the gym so you want a program that can help you get more done in less time in the gym or at home – your program should be designed to suit you.

ACTIONS SPEAKS LOUDER THAN WORDS

Everything you have read in this book until now is all knowledge. Though some people believe knowledge is power, the true power of knowledge lies in its application. You can have the right idea in your head about doing something but until you physically apply that idea it is but a good idea. Thoughts become things but for those things to become reality, action needs to be taken. Everything I have achieved in my life is as a result of acting. For me, learning something new has never been enough. Applying that knowledge, practising it, and seeing how it works has helped change my life in so many ways.

When Stephen lost 50 kilograms of body fat, I printed a poster to celebrate his milestone achievement. The poster was to be pasted on one of the walls in my gym. I asked Stephen for a caption. What would he like me to say to describe his achievement? He told me a saying that he lives by – one that has been responsible for most, if not all, of his life's achievements. He said: 'Action Speaks Louder Than Words.'

NOBODY WAS BORN A RUNNER

As a personal trainer and gym owner, sometimes I hear clients or members say, 'I am not a runner'. And to justify their point, they may add, 'I have never been a runner even from when I was young at school'.

The truth is, no one was born with a tag around their neck saying they are a runner, swimmer, cyclist, weightlifter, gym-goer, non-gym-goer, basketball player, rugby player, cricketer – you get my point. While it's true that some people are naturally gifted and some may even have the 'right genes' for certain sports, the bottom line is we all came into this world knowing nothing. Everything is learned, and through hard work, dedication, and persistence we become good at whatever it is we want to do. I say this to athletes I have trained and do train all the time: hard work always beats talent when talent does not work hard.

Yes, you may not be good at running, cycling, reading, writing – you name it. But if you apply effort, if you try hard and be consistent with it, you can get good at anything, even exercising and working out. I sometimes hear people say: 'The gym is not my thing.' Personally, I do not go to the gym because it is 'my thing'. I go to the gym because building strong bones and muscles, being fit and healthy with an abundance of energy to run around with my kids and spend quality time with my wife is my thing. I go to the gym because being in the best physical and mental shape of my life is my thing. Not the gym. The gym is just somewhere I go to make sure I get those benefits. So, though the gym may not be your thing, or you may not be a gym person, you can still do it for you, your quality of life, and for those around you.

Exercise is for everyone, and I mean *everyone*. Nobody was born a runner. So, you can become one if you want to.

CORRECT TECHNIQUE AND FORM

It is not how much you lift but how well you lift it. Having the right technique or form is very important because not only will you work your muscles better, it helps you to avoid injuries. It is a sure way to fast track your results.

In 2018 I had a young university student who visited my gym. He was visiting his parents in Mackay for a month. Being a determined gym-goer, he decided to join the gym for a month while he was here to keep working on his goals. Not only did he join the gym, he booked a session with me to write him a program as well as critique his lifting technique and form. I noticed that his technique and form with some exercises were completely off, and if he continued that way, it would take him a long time to achieve the results he wanted. And not only that, he was not too far away from injuring himself.

So, I decided to correct his form, but not without some resistance from him. Correcting his form meant he would have to drop the amount of weight he was lifting with bad form to a weight that he could lift safely with correct technique. I explained to him what I always tell every client of mine – that it is never how much you lift in the gym that matters but how well you lift it. I told him that 'form over weight' every day was the key. He then told me his real motivation for lifting heavier weights than he could safely lift was peer pressure. His friends at university were all lifting the same way, and he did not want to seem like the weakling among them. I said if he followed what I told him, it would be a short-term sacrifice for a long-term gain. Though reluctant, he decided to take heed.

When his month was up, he came to me and said, 'Thank you so much! It was hard for me to change the way I have been used to, to follow what you said, but I stuck to it and I have seen the results. I have gained an inch on my chest and I have increased my strength with the majority of my lifts.' I could see the excitement in his eyes; he was incredibly happy with his progress. One month may not have seemed like a long time, but this young man was so determined that he was coming to the gym once or twice a day on five or six days per week! 'How Bad Do You Want It?' Right?

You'll find an explanation of correct techniques for many popular exercises in appendix B.

HOW TO GET MORE DONE IN LESS TIME

All over the modern world, one of the major reasons people give for not exercising is the lack of time. We are busier these days than we ever were. We work long hours, spend more time in traffic, and even with the advancement in technology, we have not been able to get more time back for ourselves. We now spend more time on social media, glued to our phones, and watching Netflix than we make time to exercise. And one of the reasons, to be honest, is that exercise is hard. And we humans often like the path of least resistance. It is in our DNA. If something is easy, like watching TV and spending time on our phones, we do it in a heartbeat, but if it seems challenging, often we avoid it. And that is why most times even with the best intentions in mind, with our gym bags in our cars, we head home after work instead of going to the gym as we planned.

Everything is fast today; we basically want tomorrow's results yesterday. We drive fast cars, eat fast foods, crave fast internet speeds. We expect things the easy and fast way. And as a result, something as important as exercise that requires time gets seen as a burden instead of the magic pill that it is to help us live our best lives.

Considering the above, I have designed some exercise programs to help you get the most work done within the least amount of time possible so that you can carry on with your busy life and live it effectively. You'll find these in appendix C. And the way to do that is to perform:

- **Compound exercises** – these are exercises that work multiple muscle groups by moving through multiple joints and different ranges of motions. Common examples are:
  - squats
  - deadlifts
  - bench press
  - chin-ups/pull-ups
  - lunges.
- **Body weight** – these are exercises that work your entire body all at once at any given time. Common examples are:
  - burpees
  - plank
  - push ups
  - bear crawls
  - jumping jacks/star jumps.
- **Circuits** – doing multiple exercises, usually three or more, back to back for a set time or reps before having a break.
- **Super sets** – doing two sets of different exercises, usually targeting the same muscle group back to back before having a break.

Periodisation is simply planning your workouts so that you are not doing the same thing every day; in other words, so you are not working the same muscle groups every day, and even if you are, it is making sure that you are not working them to the same level of intensity. We have two broad types of skeletal muscle fibres in our body:

- slow twitch, which are used – for example – for long distance running

- fast twitch, which has three subtypes, and are usually what we use when we lift weights, sprint or do explosive exercises like jumping.

So, for example: one day you might use your slow twitch muscles – low resistance, high volume – and do some cardio, and another day you might do some strength work, and another day you might do some explosive, high-intensity plyometric workouts. Understanding this and using it to your advantage will save you hours spent working out. It also helps to keep things varied and interesting.

The exercise programs will help you boost your energy level, look and feel great about yourself, strengthen your bones and muscles, reduce stress, and be proud knowing that you are setting good examples for the people around you. And it can all be done within the shortest amount of time possible. Sometimes when it comes to exercise, it's not how long you spend exercising that matters, but how well you do it and how consistently.

STEP 5

NAIL YOUR HABITS

SO YOU CAN LIVE AN EFFECTIVE LIFE

WHAT *IS* A HABIT?

According to the Cambridge Dictionary, a 'habit is something you do regularly and often, sometimes without knowing that you are doing it', so much so that it becomes an automatic response to certain situations in life. Habits are generally formed as a means for our brains to save effort. And that is why, for example, you do not have to learn how to read again even if your last book before this one was months or even years ago.

The problem with habits, though, is that the brain cannot distinguish between a *good* habit – like working out three or more times per week – and a bad one – like consuming more than one standard drink of alcohol three or more times per week. So, if we practise good habits, they become a part of us, and so too do bad habits. Habits play such a huge role in our lives that they shape our identity. They define our being. Because habits are little things that we do each day, we do not really appreciate their magnitude until years later when we look back and realise the person we have become as a result of our habits. The saying 'big things come in little packages' is absolutely true, and it is so with habits too.

If we practise little good habits everyday, over time the outcome is huge, and it shapes our lives for good. On the other hand, if we practise bad habits, they compound over time and it changes our lives for the worse. Let's take for example the documentary *Super Size Me*, in which Morgan Spurlock, an American independent filmmaker, ate nothing but McDonald's for 30 days, three times a day – trying everything on the menu. At the end of 30 days, he gained 10.8 kilograms. And that was just for 30 days! Imagine what the outcome would be for – say – a year, two years, or even five years. Now, nobody is going to eat McDonald's for every meal every day, but this does show the dramatic effect in a short space of time of the habit of eating poorly.

For the majority of us it may not be that drastic. But when I look at our beautiful country Australia, unfortunately more than 60%

of our adult population today is overweight or obese. We did not get here in one day. We got here as result of our habits. And by no means am I trying to shame anyone – I'm trying to help provide a solution; to help us identify the habits that could be the cause of our problems – weight gain, sleepless nights, low energy levels and low productivity – as well as become aware of the ones that help us live our best lives – regular exercise, making the right food choices – and continuing to do them or to form new ones.

When it comes to the subject of habits, there are three great books that I highly recommend reading: *The 7 Habits of Highly Effective People* by Stephen R. Covey, *Atomic Habits* by James Clear, and *The Power of Habits* by Charles Duhigg. These books will help you understand habits on a deeper level: personal, organisational as well as culturally, how habits are formed, and how to break bad habits and form new ones.

For the purpose of this book my focus will be on habits relating to your health and wellbeing, and I will also talk about how you can break bad habits and form new and beneficial ones.

TAKING RESPONSIBILITY

There comes a time in our lives when we all must take responsibility for ourselves and realise that no one else or anything else is responsible for the situations we may be facing as a result of the decisions or lack of decisions we made. Everything that happens to us in life – good or bad – happens for a reason. It's our responsibility then to find that reason. To make sense of it and to identify the meaning behind it. One of my favourite quotations of all time, and one that has had such a profound impact on my life since discovering it, is from Viktor Frankl, an Austrian neurologist and psychiatrist who also happened to be a holocaust survivor. Viktor states:

> Between stimulus and response there is a space. In that space is our power to choose our response. In our response lies our growth and our freedom.

Viktor's book *Man's Search for Meaning* chronicles his life as an inmate in Nazi concentration camps, where he was beaten, tortured, and worked to the brink of death in unimaginable conditions. His wife, father, mother, and brother all died in the camps. Despite those horrific, dehumanised experiences, he found meaning and became a world-renowned neurologist and psychiatrist.

At this point, you are probably wondering, what has Viktor Frankl got to do with me? Quite frankly, the answer is nothing, but the quote above has everything to do with helping you take responsibility for the situations in your life right now. This book is all about helping you live your best life – how you can have more energy and vitality so that you can be more productive during your working day, as well as when you get home to be able to spend quality time with your family or loved ones. It is also about how you can develop a physique that when you look in the mirror you can be happy with, as well as being happy knowing you are setting good examples for the people around you. To be able to achieve all these things and more, you must first identify where you find yourself right now, what decisions led you there, and make a conscious effort to take responsibility for your life and make meaningful change.

I was born in a country that went through 14 years of civil war. At a young age, I was separated from family, I lost close friends and relatives, and found myself going from one refugee camp to another. Looking back at my life in those refugee camps and looking at my life now, sometimes I ask myself, *how did I end up here?* It still feels surreal and like a miracle. Being surrounded by all those hopeless and helpless situations, it was easy – and understandable – for anybody to give up. And many people did. But in life we can either sit down and wish for our life to change or we can get up and change it. Even though not having a job was the norm, I chose to not be a part of that norm – I sought employment. Even though you could be forgiven for not caring about making a difference, I co-founded a literacy program to help kids and adults learn how to read and write.

Even though the thought of where my next meal was going to come from dominated every day, I still sought personal development and did my best each day to improve, and part of that decision led me to Australia today.

You have the power

My point is, if Viktor Frankl, despite all that he went through, could choose his response to the situations he was dealt and find meaning in his existence, anyone can. If I too – on a totally different level to Viktor – can go from worrying about where my next meal was going to come from, going days without food, and wondering where my family was, to being in the position today where I can write this book for you to read, you too can find meaning in whatever situation you may be facing right now and make the choice to get up and change it. You have the power to choose the response to the situations specific to you and find meaning in the suffering.

We need to take responsibility for our lives and turn every negative situation into a positive one. I get it: life can be cruel, and sometimes it is not even your fault that negative things happen to you. But always remember you have the power to choose how you *respond* to those situations. Your response will either bring about your growth and freedom or the opposite.

Here is another example. In 2020, the world as we knew it changed forever. The coronavirus pandemic spread from China and wreaked havoc across the globe. Many lost lives and livelihoods, and economies around the world collapsed. Everyone felt the effects of the virus, including myself. In an attempt to 'flatten the curve', our government imposed lockdown restrictions which, unfortunately, meant that I had to shut the doors to my gyms. It was a devastating feeling – one that is extremely hard to put into words.

Here is some background as to why this was really painful. Prior to the coronavirus pandemic, in 2019 our goal was to expand our gym so that we could reach and cater for more everyday people.

Finding the right building at a price we could afford caused a great deal of stress. I looked at several options with no success.

While in the middle of instructing one of our 9am Muscle Garden classes one day, I had a missed call which was followed by a text message from the leasing manager of one of the major shopping centres here in Mackay about putting our gym in their centre. It was a surprise to me because when I first started Muscle Garden, out of curiosity I inquired about what it would cost to have a gym in that very centre, and I was told that they did not allow gyms. So you can imagine my surprise when I read the message. Anyway, I met with the leasing manager and the shopping centre manager, who conveyed to me that our reputation in town and family-oriented values aligned with their shopping centre, which provided a space for families to shop, dine, and be entertained. I thought that this was a compliment, a sign that what we were doing and who we are was being noticed.

After a couple of months of negotiations, we arrived at a deal that appeared to be a win/win for us and the shopping centre. But there was a condition. For me to have the agreed floor space, they had to relocate an existing tenant. With this in mind, I knew the deal could go either way. So, I kept looking at other options. I took responsibility for the situation and acted proactively.

Unfortunately, that tenant did not see it as in their best interest to relocate, but it did not matter much because by this time I had already found another location – the one we are in now. I did not stop searching, hoping that the deal with the shopping centre would fall in my favour. And when it did not work out, I never blamed the tenant who refused to move, or the shopping centre. That tenant was doing what was best for them, as I was trying to do for my business.

Although we did not end up in that shopping centre, the experience taught me a lot – knowledge that I would later apply in negotiating with the leasing manager of another shopping centre where we now have our second gym in Marian.

The truth is we did not go into 2019 with the plan to open a second gym; the thought did not even cross my mind, but that was exactly what we did. So, you can see now why having to close due to the pandemic was especially painful, given the time and effort that had just gone into opening the new locations both in Marian and in Mackay.

Taking responsibility and acknowledging we are where we are today because of our choices or lack of choices, our decisions or lack of decisions, and owning that we had a part to play in it all is a first step to truly achieving change.

BEING PROACTIVE

We need to be proactive about our health and wellness. Being proactive is simply taking charge, creating, or controlling the outcome of a situation *before* it happens, instead of responding to it *after* it has happened. In my line of work, even though I do see clients who make proactive decisions about their health and wellbeing, unfortunately the majority of the time when I see them it is because they have 'let themselves go'. Proactive decisions would be not waiting until something is wrong before you go to see a doctor or a personal trainer. They would be getting regular blood tests done to see what's going on with your body, doing your biannual check-ups at the dentist so your teeth stay healthy, checking your moles regularly so they do not turn into melanoma, and doing regular exercise at least three times per week to stay fit and healthy.

If being proactive is taking charge, creating, or controlling the outcome of a situation before it happens instead of just responding to it after it has happened, then being reactive is the opposite of that. Being reactive is *not* taking charge, creating, or controlling the outcome of a situation before it happens. It is simply waiting for something to happen and then responding to it. Being reactive is waiting until you are overweight before doing something about it, or even worse, it is waiting until being overweight or obese leads to diabetes or some other weight-related illnesses before deciding to do something about it.

Being proactive is about preventing, and being reactive is about curing. And as we know, prevention is always better than cure. Take control of your life. Make proactive decisions and not reactive ones. Do not wait until your weight or health is in the unhealthy range before you do something about it. Do something about it now. Do not wait until you are sick before you see the doctor. Do regular check-ups, do regular exercise to strengthen you heart, bones, and muscles. Do not say, 'It's raining so I'm not going for a run'. Say, 'I planned to go for a run, and regardless of the rain, I will still go'. By so doing you will also strengthen your willpower.

Even though some people tend to be more proactive and others more reactive, I do not want to use the phrase 'proactive or reactive people' because at any given point in time we can all choose to be either proactive or reactive. Those who are more reactive can learn to be more proactive. It takes practice. You will have to become aware of your situation and ask yourself, 'Am I being proactive or reactive? And will this choice yield the best outcome?' For example: while being proactive is making sure that you are not overweight in the first place, you can react to the situation by making sure you do not go from being overweight to obese – which then would be a proactive decision to not be obese. When clients come to see me because they have waited until something has gone wrong, I still applaud them for doing something about it because in their reactive decision to do something about their health and wellbeing lies a proactive decision to not let the situation get any worse than what it already is.

Choose to be proactive in all things that you do, and you will create for yourself the life that you want to live.

VISUALISING YOUR DESIRED RESULT

Before a new client comes onboard as a personal training client, I usually sit down with them for a consultation, and here are some of the questions I ask them:

- 'At the end of your training sessions what outcome do you hope to achieve?'

- 'What does the end look like for you? Can you please describe it to me?'

- 'What does it feel like to be in that position?'

- 'What would it mean to you if you achieved that result?'

- 'What are your emotions if you were in that position right now?'

- 'How does it change your life? Is it for the better or worse?'

- 'Who are the people around you that are going to benefit from you achieving your desired end goal?'

The reason I ask these questions is to help my clients create a noticeably clear mental and physical picture of what they want. The clearer the goal, and the emotions that are attached to that goal, the more likely they are to achieve it.

Visualisation is an especially important habit that I use all the time. I remember when I signed up my heaviest client ever. I was excited and nervous at the same time. I was nervous because I had not trained someone his size before, but I was also very excited because I visualised this client being a completely different person if he stuck to the training. And indeed, he went on to lose a lot of body fat, build lean muscle mass, and went from being an unhealthy person to a healthy one.

Before I set out to do something, I first visualise what it is going to be. The purpose of doing that is to figure out what the end is going to look like and then begin with that end in mind – if the end is indeed a desired one. I usually picture what I want my life, family, and business to look like, and then I start with that end image in mind and work backwards until it becomes reality.

What is your desired end result? What do you picture your health to be like? If you were a perfect physical specimen five years from now, what would that look like? Make a habit of visualising your end result or goal and start from there and work backwards.

PRIORITISING YOUR HEALTH

Have you ever heard the saying, 'Your health is your wealth'? And have you sat down and really thought about what it means? If not, well now might be a good time to do so. It is quite a cliché and one that is taken for granted. But our health is indeed our wealth, and it should not come at the mercy of other things.

Unfortunately, these days, in this fast-paced world, it is really the opposite. We trade our health for wealth, not really considering the consequences. The Dalai Lama, when asked what surprised him most about humanity, answered:

> Man. Because he sacrifices his health in order to make money. Then he sacrifices money to recuperate his health. And then he is so anxious about the future that he does not enjoy the present; the result being that he does not live in the present or the future; he lives as if he is never going to die and then dies having never really lived.

Wow! The first time I read this, I was astounded. It was during a difficult period in my business and family life, a time in which I was trading my hours for dollars. I could not afford to be away from work, and I also could not stomach being away from my wife and son Malachi when he was first born. I felt trapped. Mentally and physically I was exhausted. But there comes a time when we all must sit down and ask ourselves, *what is really important?* That was the journey I went on which changed everything for me, the business, and my family.

You could have all the material wealth in the world, but what use is it if you are lying in a hospital and cannot enjoy it, or don't really have the energy to do anything? Having good health comprises both sound mental health and physical health. When you are in the best physical and mental shape of your life, you feel unstoppable. You feel like you are on top of the world, even if you do not have all the material wealth in the world. You are more content and grateful for the things you have, instead of the things you do not. You have a clear mind, and plenty of energy and vitality to live your best life.

Our body is the only vehicle we have to navigate through this thing called life, and how you treat your body determines how you go through life. Unlike cars, our bodies are not just about getting from point A to point B. It is about *how well* we get from point A to point B. In our right mind we would not put diesel in a car that runs on petrol, but unfortunately that is how most of us treat our bodies. The majority of people on this planet today, especially in the western world where everyone is trying to get ahead in a rat race, are just existing. We are not really living. Instead of being a 'human being' we are a 'human doing'. And most of the time it comes at the expense of both our mental and physical health.

More and more people are taking stress leave today. Prioritising your health would mean you do not wait until you get to that point. Today there are more people suffering from burnouts, mental health problems as well as physical health issues – you do not have to be one of them. Prioritise your health and you will have the greatest wealth ever known.

HOW HABITS ARE FORMED

As previously mentioned in this step, habits are formed as a means for our brains to save effort. When a habit becomes automatic, our brains to a degree switch off, in the sense that we can perform that habit without even thinking about it. Take learning a new skill. At first it seems overwhelming. You feel like there are too many steps involved, the process is taking too long, and there is too much to think about. You even sometimes get frustrated and think about giving up. But after you successfully learn that skill, with enough practice, it becomes a habit. You now perform that skill or habit automatically with so much ease. Some would even say, 'I can do it with my eyes closed'. When I teach clients to do a squat or a deadlift for the first time, sometimes they do not pick up the information I give them and the demonstration I show them right away. For some it seems impossible. But with continuous practice, they perform what seemed impossible at first with so much ease that they do not even remember it being that hard to start with. For a habit to form, it must be repeated enough times that it becomes automatic.

Stephen R. Covey, in his groundbreaking book *The 7 Habits of Highly Effective People*, defines habits as the intersection of:

- knowledge – knowing *what* to do and *why*

- skill – knowing *how* to do it

- desire – having the *motivation*, the *want* to do it.

Knowing what to do and why is not enough. Many people know they need to exercise and eat healthily and why they need to do so, but if they do not know how to do it, a habit will not form. And even if they know how to exercise and eat healthily, if they do not have the motivation or the want to do it, a habit will not form. According to Covey, the knowledge, skill and desire must all fall into place to facilitate habit formation.

Charles Duhigg in his book *The Power of Habits* describes a habit loop that is responsible for how habits are formed. It is a three-step process called Cue, Routine and Reward. Cue is what triggers the habit to get the reward, routine is the habit you perform to get to the reward, and the reward is the satisfaction you get as a result of performing that habit, and it is also what makes the habit automatic.

James Clear in his book *Atomic Habits* also describes a habit loop, which he refers to as the backbone for how habits are formed.

He describes a four-step pattern of Cue, Craving, Response, and Reward. Cue is the trigger to act, craving is the motivation or desire to act, response is your action, and reward is the end goal.

Let's look at an example. Although I am a very disciplined person in the majority of areas in my life, like everybody, I am not perfect. I formed a habit that I am not proud of, and one that I have been working to get rid of, and truthfully am now better at. When I am in my car driving and my phone buzzes, I feel the urge to check the message. But I understand it is risky and illegal to check my phone while I drive. So, most times I wait until I get to a traffic light, and when the light is red, I quickly check my phone. I did not realise how automatic this process was until I decided to stop it. My cue was the phone buzzing, routine was me being in my car driving and stopping at a traffic light. The reward was reaching to my passenger seat and grabbing my phone and checking the content of the message.

In another sense, cue equals phone buzzing, craving equals me dying to find out what caused the phone to buzz, response is me picking up the phone once I was at a red light, and the reward is finding out who messaged and what their message was about.

This I found had become so automatic that my phone did not even have to buzz for me to want to check it. Between where I live and where I work is a 3.6 kilometre route. There are four traffic lights along the way. Every time I got to a traffic light, out of habit, I reached out for my phone in my passenger seat. I found I could ignore my phone buzzing, but the minute I saw a traffic light, and especially when it turned red, that was my cue and my habit was reaching for my phone. And because I traversed those traffic lights multiple times per day, I had the endless temptation of practising that habit. But I decided to break this habit because it is something I did not want to be doing.

So, how do you break a bad habit?

HOW TO BREAK BAD HABITS

To break a bad habit, you must first identify what triggers the habit. What happens immediately before you perform the habit? Identify clearly what the habit is. What is the routine, and what is the reward? What satisfaction do you get as a result of performing that habit? Once you have clearly identified the habit loop then you can put in measures to change – something I am going to talk about shortly in this step.

The truth is, no one sets out with the intention of developing a bad habit. I certainly never woke up one day and decided: I am going develop a habit of checking my phone every time I stop at a traffic light. Phones have become a part of our lives very much today; we do not only receive and make phone calls on them anymore, we now do banking on our phones, watch videos, movies, and TV shows, read or listen to books on them and study, as well as do social media – Facebook, Twitter, Instagram … you name it. With all the power and the distractions that come with our phones today, it is easy to become glued to them. Parents are now even using digital screens to keep their kids entertained while they carry out other tasks. No parent ever gives their children digital screens with the intention for their children to get addicted to them. But as numerous studies show today, that is exactly what is happening. Kids are becoming screen addicts. And I must say that while it is true some technology is good for children, too much of anything may not be so good.

So, whether your bad habit is checking your phone while driving, eating junk food, saying to yourself you are not good enough, procrastinating and being lazy, spending too much time on social media, avoiding exercise, or making excuses, all these habits can be broken.

But once a habit is formed, we must understand that it is extremely hard to break. Good or bad, all habits serve us in some way, and that is why we do them. Our brain releases a chemical called dopamine which is a neurotransmitter; in other words, it is a messenger which is responsible for carrying out communication between nerve cells within the nervous system. Dopamine plays a major role in our reward-motivated behaviour and is most commonly associated with the brain's pleasure and reward system. So, when I am driving and I stop at a red light, a message is sent among nerve cells in my brain which triggers the craving for me to check my phone. And if I respond by checking my phone, I get the reward. It is also part of the reason why some people cannot walk past a donut shop without eating one. Just the smell of it triggers a response. We often respond to the cues that give us the greatest pleasure and reward, and this is why it's so easy to form a bad habit – the reward, unlike a good habit, is instant.

So! How do you break a bad habit?

Make it hard to access

Once you have identified what causes the habit that you are trying to break, your next action is to take it out of sight and make it hard to access. The old adage 'out of sight, out of mind' works wonders when it comes to breaking bad habits or habits that do not serve us positively in the long term. With my habit of checking my phone every time I came to a red light, the best thing to do will be to get rid of the temptation. Since I cannot remove every traffic light or take a different route that does not have a traffic light, I can make my phone hard to get to. So, what I did to help me break the habit was I put my phone in the enclosed centre console of my car, or sometimes I threw it in the back seat. The first time I did this I was amazed at how automatic my habit of reaching for my phone the moment I approached a set of traffic lights had become. I was reaching for my phone without even thinking about it, and when it wasn't even there. The second I saw the light going from amber to red, that was my cue.

When I reached for my phone at the first set of traffic lights on my way home and realised that I had placed it in the centre console, I thought this would have been enough to remind me at the next traffic light that my phone was not on my passenger seat where I could easily reach over and grab it. But this habit had become so automatic that I reached for my phone at all three remaining traffic lights. I was so blown away that when I got home, I could not wait to share the story with my wife. That is how habits control our lives.

Change the way you look at it: focus on the negatives

If you ask any non-smoker what they think about smoking, their initial response would often be, 'It's disgusting', followed by, 'Yuck'. Now, what do you think are the chances of someone who views smoking cigarettes in this manner ever becoming a smoker? You guessed it: none. What if we looked at our bad habits the way a non-smoker views smoking?

In 2009 when I first moved to Australia, it became noticeably clear to me that drinking alcohol was very much a huge part of the Aussie culture. It was impossible to not have alcohol at every social event. I remember I would go out with my group of mates and sometimes I would drink until I was completely 'blind' or 'wasted' – words I had not associated with drinking before. That was the norm. In 2010 I lived with a housemate who would drink a glass or two of wine every night with dinner. And whenever I was home for dinner, I would also share a bottle of wine with him. It became a habit.

When I moved out, the habit stayed with me. I moved into a house with a group of housemates who were also colleagues and they did not mind their drinking either. It was like a party every weekend. My habit of drinking went from one or two glasses per night with dinner to a bottle, and sometimes two bottles. I consistently drank at least one bottle of wine every night for about six months. I would order wine by the cartoon to keep in my room, or run down to Dan Murphy's which was just down the road from where we lived whenever I ran out of wine.

In 2011, a year out from when I started Muscle Garden Personal Training, I decided to quit drinking on my birthday of that year. I figured if I was going to help people live a healthy life through exercise and nutrition then I needed to set a good example for them to follow. I had to change my identity. My new identity became, *I am a non-drinker – I do not drink alcohol*. I changed the way I looked at drinking alcohol all together. It went from being something that many, including myself, perceived as a cool and fun thing to do, to 'this could give a client the wrong impression'; 'I am not setting a good example if I continue to drink'; 'they may not take me seriously'.

Quitting drinking was not because I wanted or expected my clients to do the same. No. It was quite simply that I wanted to lead by example. I wanted to set a standard for my clients that if they ever wanted to stop drinking, they could use me as an example that it was possible. And what helped me quit drinking was changing the way I looked at it. I did not see it as cool anymore. I did not see it as fun anymore. I remember there was a trainer I knew who went to the gym where I trained at the time, and whenever I would see him up town drunk, he would say to me, 'Do as I say, not as I do'. Each to their own, but I knew that was not the kind of trainer I wanted to be and it helped me in the way I looked at drinking.

After I quit drinking, some friends would say to me, 'You are no fun'. It did not matter, because even without alcohol I believed I was still having more fun than they were. I could enter into any room and, without trying, I would easily be the loudest. I told myself I did not need alcohol to have fun and, quite frankly, that is the truth. If you want to break a bad habit, change the way look at that habit.

Have an accountability partner or group

Having an accountability partner or group works wonders, especially if they are likeminded people who will hold you to a high standard. It's part of the reason why Alcoholics Anonymous has been so successful. And there have been many studies to prove why having an accountability partner or group works.

Being a part of an accountability group helped me in writing the first 34,000 words of this book in just six weeks. At the writing of this book, I am a member of two accountability groups. As humans, we value the opinions of others, especially about what they think of us, and most times we would do anything to avoid the feeling of being a letdown. And this feeling of not letting the team down or being a disappointment alone drives us to perform.

In 2018 I ran my first online 8 Week Body Transformation Challenge, and 55 members of my gym signed up for the challenge. The challenge was phenomenally successful, with a remarkably high completion rate. During the challenge we had our highest gym attendance record up to that time. Part of the reason the challenge was so successful was the accountability groups – something most participants said was the best part of the challenge. I split all 55 members into five accountability groups. In their separate groups they had to look out for each other and hold each other to a very high standard. They had to do their workouts and change the habits that were not going to help them achieve the results they wanted from doing the challenge. And there was a friendly competition between accountability groups. For a group to win, each member of that group had to commit not only to their personal success but the overall success of their group. I saw groups getting together to do their workouts, they were catching up for coffee, new friendships and new training buddies were formed. Even after the challenge had finished these members were still getting together to train and continue on with some of the habits they had picked up from the challenge.

As a personal trainer, one of the reasons I find personal training to be so successful is because of the accountability it creates. If you just tell yourself, 'I will go to the gym to train', unless you are really motivated, the chances of you not getting there are higher compared to if you had a personal training session booked with a trainer. As part of my personal training agreement, there is an accountability clause stating that if they need to cancel their session they must do it outside of 24 hours before the session, and if not, they will be charged the full cost of the session. And I also add that if they cancel multiple times, their personal training agreement would be terminated as it would be a waste of their money and my time. Sometimes

I use my discretion and do not charge them if they could not make the session due to an unforeseen circumstance, but what that clause does is it reduces the number of times clients cancel. It holds them accountable.

Even with my online training app where I do not train clients in person, there is an area on the app where they must record that they have done the exercise and record their weight and number of sets they have performed. This creates accountability, and they get a small win from logging their workouts.

Whether it's your husband or wife, friend or colleague, personal trainer, coach, or mentor, if you want to break a bad habit, get an accountability partner or group that will hold you to a high standard.

HOW TO DEVELOP GOOD HABITS

What we refer to as good habits are those habits that serve us for the better long term. They are the ones that benefit us in the future. And that is part of the reason why it is so difficult to form good habits. Unlike bad habits, usually the reward is delayed, and so sometimes it takes effort to form them. For example: you can start exercising today and you might not see results right away. It could take you a month, 3, 6, or even 12 months before you see the results you want.

One of the first questions people always ask me before they sign up for personal training is, 'How long will it take before I start seeing results?' As previously mentioned, we do not necessarily perform a habit because we like the habit itself but because of the reward we get from it. Good habits take time to form – they are the consistent accumulation of small efforts towards that habit over a period of time. Bad habits, on the other hand, do not require as much effort and the rewards are instant. For example: if you get a craving for sugar and you eat a block of chocolate, you get the instant reward. If you want to lose weight and be healthy, you have to exercise and eat healthily, and the results will take time. One fundamental rule to remember about habit formation is that what gives you instant reward now may not always be good for you long term, and what gives you a delayed reward may be good for you in the long run.

While it is true that good habits may not give us instant rewards, there are things we can do to make the experience worthwhile and enjoyable, like putting in place measures and tracking systems. A common example would be writing this book. Getting up at an average time of 3am most mornings to write may not be rewarding at the time, but having a tracker on my phone to see how many days per week I stick to my writing schedule and word count gives me that reward, and it makes the process enjoyable to see that I am making progress. The trick is to do something that gives you a reward for doing a good habit without feeling like it is a burden or that you are missing out.

A bad example of this method is what is often referred to as a 'cheat day'. Though widely popular in the fitness world today, it is something that does not make sense to me. Eating junk food one day a week because you have spent the other days eating well and exercising is not a vote in favour of the habit you are trying to form or the person you are trying to become. A better reward could be a new outfit to fit into once you have lost some weight as a result of eating healthily and exercising, or new workout gear or a massage for sticking to your routine of exercising and eating healthily. The point is, whatever you choose to use to reward yourself for performing a good habit or staying away from a bad one should be in line with that habit you are trying to form or break as well as the person you want to become or the identity you are trying to form.

So, how do we form a good habit?

Make it easy to access

If rule number one for breaking a bad habit is to make it hard to access then rule number one for forming a good habit is the opposite of that. One excellent example of this comes from the supermarkets. Supermarkets use what is called a 'planogram', which means a diagram or model that indicates where retail products are placed on shelves to maximise sales. Take one guess where the best location is. If you guessed 'eye level', you would be correct.

When something is placed in our line of sight and it is easy to get to, 9 times out of 10, being human, we will take the path of least resistance. We do not like to bend down or reach up high to grab an item unless we do not have a choice. And this is something we can use to our advantage when forming good habits.

We can use a planogram to maximise our odds for performing good habits. So, for example: if you want to get into the habit of exercising, have your workout clothes out the night before and put them in a place where you can easily see and access them. I know some people who even go to bed in their workout gear so that when they get up in the morning they are ready to go! If you want to get into the habit of eating healthily, buy healthy meals, fill your fridge with healthy snacks, and surround yourself with healthy food. If you want to get into the habit of reading, put a book beside your bedside table. A little while ago I wanted my wife to read Dale Carnegie's book *How to Win Friends and Influence People*. She is not a big fan of non-fiction. So, without saying a word, I put it on her bedside table.

She ignored the book for the first week or two, but eventually she picked it up and read it. It was the first thing she saw each morning when she woke up, and the last thing she saw each night before she went to sleep. It was in her line of sight and it was easy to access.

If you want to form a good habit, make it easy for yourself. Reduce the friction.

Change the way you look at it: focus on the positives

If rule number 2 for breaking a bad habit is to change the way you look at it by focusing on the negative aspects of that habit, then rule number 2 for forming a good a habit is the opposite – change the way you look at the habit by pointing out the positive aspects of that habit. As previously mentioned, good habits are hard habits. Unlike bad habits, they do take time and effort. And being humans who naturally gravitate to the path of least resistance, we sometimes avoid a good habit. But if we can learn to change the way we look at a good habit and focus on its long-term benefits and how it is going to change our lives and the lives of our loved ones or people around us, it helps to make forming a good habit or breaking a bad one easier.

Many times I have clients come in to see me to change their lives because they want to be able to run around with their children. They want to have an abundance of energy and vitality, to not only be productive at work but also at home. They want to be able to look in the mirror and be happy with what they see. They want to be good role models for the people around them. Usually one way that I use to help them get there is through exercise and proper nutrition, none of which is easy, but the benefits of being able to run around with their children, to be in their best physical and mental shape, and know that they are setting good examples for loved ones, far outweigh the pain and heartache of exercising and eating healthily.

One common example I use when it comes to changing the way we look at a good habit which is hard is burpees. I believe about 98% of the fitness world hates burpees. And I do not blame them. Burpees are hard; in fact, ridiculously hard. A burpee is a full-body exercise that involves you taking your whole body to the ground then getting back up and jumping in the air, all in one motion. But if you only look at the pain from doing burpees and the fact that you do not really see an immediate reward from doing them, you may not like them.

I did an experiment in 2019 where for the whole month of March, I ran a challenge called the Mackay March Burpee Challenge. Close to 50 people put their hand up to do the challenge. For every day in March, the participants had to do a minute of burpees, and it did not matter the type of burpees or number of reps they performed. They just had to commit to doing burpees each day for 31 days. Out of the almost 50 people who signed up for the challenge, guess how many completed it? Two! Including me!

So, what if there was another way to look at burpees so it was not perceived as an all-pain-and-no-gain exercise? The way I see it, burpees represent the challenges we face in life. To perform a burpee, you must go down to the ground and come back up and jump in the air, all in one motion. To me it is the representation that it does not matter how many times life knocks you down to the ground – what matters is the ability to get back up each time. You never finish a burpee lying on the ground. You always find a way to get back up onto your own two feet. So, if I do not have the mental and physical capacity to handle burpees, how am I supposed to handle life – family, business, and all the other challenges that life throws at us?

If you want to form a good habit, change the way you look at it – find meaning in the suffering.

Have an accountability partner or group that is on the same path as you

An accountability partner or group can help you break a bad habit in the same way that they can help you form a good one. Find someone or a group that is on the same path as you. For example, if you are trying to quit smoking or drinking, hanging around people who drink or smoke all the time may not be your best option. On the other hand, if you are trying to quit drinking alcohol then Alcoholics Anonymous may be a good option. It is one accountability group that has been around for years, with a proven track record of success for its members.

How and why Alcoholics Anonymous works so well has defied science for many years. When we are put in an environment with likeminded people who are on the same journey as we are and the culture of that environment is geared towards success, we have no choice but contribute to the overall success of the group, even if it means doing something we do not want to do. Our own personal success then becomes less important than the success of the group. But when we find ourselves in a group where the standards are low then we become the product of that association. Say, for example, you are a member of a fitness group that encourages eating junk food, drinking alcohol, and partying – guess what your result is going to be? Exercise is never a green light to do all of those things. So, you may exercise all you want but if the eating and drinking habits or standards of your group do not change, you will stay the same. If you want to form a good habit, have an accountability partner or group that is on the same path as the person you want to become.

HOW TO MAKE GOOD HABITS LAST

All habits, good or bad, compound over time. Starting a habit that is too hard by jumping straight in the deep end most times will not last. So, let's see how to make good habits last:

1. **Start small.** The key to making good habits last is to start small. I remember one time my wife decided we were going vegetarian. Not that I was keen on the idea, but the way she planned on starting, I knew straight away that it would not work, so I did not even bother arguing with the lovely lady. She came out one day and said: 'We are eating vegetarian all week.' I said, 'Are you sure about that? Don't you maybe want to start with a day or two first and see how we go?' She said, 'No,' to which I replied, 'Okay, no worries.' She was determined … for two days. On the third day, I was at work and got a text message from her saying: 'Okay, I have had enough, I need meat!' I laughed.

    If you make small, positive changes each day, they shape who you are over time. Our gym appeals to everyday people. People who either have not been to the gym for a long time or have never set foot in a gym before. Usually when we assess these members, we give them a program to follow. Depending on their abilities and goals, the programs usually range anywhere from 8 to 15 repetitions of each exercise for about three to five sets. What I found was that this was sometimes overwhelming for some members, especially for those who were just starting out. So, I introduced a different method. Each new member just starting out had to start small and gradually build up with their training programs. If, for example, a program had four sets, they had to work up to that number of sets over four weeks. After the program was completed, in week one they only needed to show up, do their warmup, and do one set of everything that was on their program for that day. Then two sets in week two, three sets in week three, and four sets in week four. The idea is to first establish the habit of showing up and not having to worry about being too sore or being overwhelmed with the number of exercises. During the first week it may feel like they are not doing much, and because of this they want to come in because it means they can progress to another level. By the time they get to week four they have not only adjusted to coming to the gym, but their muscles would have also gradually adjusted and can handle the workload. In my experience, the gym members who usually do not last long are the overzealous ones who right upon signing up start training one or two times per day, five to seven days a week. Unless you are a professional athlete, that kind of workload is difficult to maintain. We can break any bad habit or start a good one by starting small and progressively building overtime. Big things really do come in small packages.

2. **Track and measure your progress.** You cannot manage what you cannot measure. And that is why it's important to know your baseline. To have an idea of where you are starting from. Armed with that information, make the conscious effort to focus on what is working and not so much on what is not. Because good habits have delayed gratification, tracking and measuring, and rewarding yourself along the way, will help you stay focused. The goal is to fall in love with the process and the results will come. You can track how many days you have worked out or how many times you have made good choices – choices that will benefit your future self over ones that do the

opposite. You can celebrate those achievements daily, weekly, monthly, quarterly, every six months, and every year. Tracking and measuring is the one habit that helps tie all your good habits together and helps you continue on until those habits become automatic. Here is a tracking process you can use:

- *Daily:* aim for at least 30 minutes of physical activity per day.

- *Weekly:* aim for at least three workouts per week.

- *Monthly:* do a body scan to see how you are progressing.

- *Quarterly:* get a program review.

- *Biannually:* see how far you have come. Reassess your goals and make sure they are in line with who you want to become.

- *Yearly:* repeat the above.

Breaking a bad habit or forming a new one is never going to be an easy task, but it helps if you have a strong reason behind it. Ask yourself, 'Who do I want to become and why?', and, 'By becoming this person, how is my life going to change and who is going to benefit as a result of my change?' Let the answers to these questions be the driving force behind the actions you take. Making a change is not going to be easy but the key is to focus on what is working. You will slip up whether you like it or not, but do not let that derail you. As long as you are not slipping up more than you are making progress, that is all that matters.

STEP 6

GET YOUR TIME BACK SO YOU CAN LIVE LIFE ON YOUR OWN TERMS

According the Old Testament book of Ecclesiastes Chapter 3 Verses 1 to 8:

1. There is a time for everything, and a season for every activity under the heavens.

2. A time to be born and a time to die, a time to plant and a time to uproot.

3. A time to kill and a time to heal, a time to tear down and a time to build.

4. A time to weep and a time to laugh, a time to mourn and a time to dance.

5. A time to scatter stones and a time to gather them, a time to embrace and a time to refrain from embracing.

6. A time to search and a time to give up, a time to keep and a time to throw away.

7. A time to tear and a time to mend, a time to be silent and a time to speak.

8. A time to love and a time to hate, a time for war and a time for peace.

As far back as time goes, even in Biblical days, the idea of time has always been a vital part of human existence. A time to hunt for food and a time to gather. Time is so important that it is regarded as the most valuable currency in the world today. We have one life to live, and how we spend our time on this earth determines the outcome of the life we lead, the legacy we leave behind, the impact we have on our loved ones, the people around us and our society as a whole.

Even though time is so vital, we live in a world today where people are so busy that they do not make time for themselves. The number one reason people say they do not exercise or do things that would benefit their health and wellbeing is because of the lack of time.

Why is this? Why is everyone so time poor?

THE AGE OF THE RAT RACE

We live in the age of the rat race, a way of life in which people are caught up in a fiercely competitive struggle for wealth or power, or both. The rat race means no life/work balance, no independence, high stress, long commutes, and general dissatisfaction with life. What this does is leave the everyday person, especially business owners, with no time for themselves because they are constantly chasing, competing, and struggling to get ahead and to be able to feed their families as well as keep a roof over their heads. They often put everyone and everything first before themselves.

When I first started Muscle Garden in 2012, this was my life. It was only work that mattered. My mindset at the time was that if I can help at least one person turn their life around by achieving their health and fitness goals, and if I can provide for myself at the same time while doing what I love, then that is all that matters. In saying that, part of the reason I went into business for myself, as previously mentioned in this book, was that – though I did not have a family at the time – when the time came, I wanted to be in the position where my wife and children would be able to come to my workplace to visit. I imagined my children running around the gym and jumping on the equipment. That was my dream. That was what I visualised. I could not see this working on a mine site. And that was the reason why, even though the money was good, it was a no-brainer leaving the mining industry.

Compounding problems

In 2013, Jessica and I decided to buy a house. Initially, we were knocked back by the banks for two reasons: firstly, I had not been in business for at least two years – a prerequisite for business owners, and secondly, we did not have enough money to pay for a deposit on a home. I walked away feeling rejected, and so I did what I always did when I faced challenges. I told myself that the next time we went to the bank for a loan to buy a house, we would make them an offer they would not say no to.

As a result of this, I buried myself in my work. As work kept getting busier, I kept saying 'yes'. I was doing 15-hour days, six days a week – public holidays and all. I was doing what I had to do to get us to where we wanted to be. My wife understood what we were working towards, so she did not complain. But I knew it affected her. She comes from a close-knit family and had lots of friends she hung out with and did things with. When she decided to move up from the Gold Coast to Mackay to be with me, she sacrificed all of that. All she had up here was me. So, for me to be working all those long hours meant that I was leaving her at home early in the morning for work and coming home late at night, and it was not easy. I remember one time someone tried to break into our house, and she decided she was not going to be at home by herself anymore. She would come to work with me early in the morning before my 5am start. Some mornings she would be curled up on one of the exercise mats on the floor in my office. Then she would get ready for her work, and then come back to the gym when she was finished and stay at the gym until I was finished work after 8pm for us to go home. We got our first dog so that she could feel safe at home.

Anyway, in 2014, less than a year after we got rejected, we applied for a loan again to buy our house that we now live in, at the writing of this book, and our application was approved. I was then in business for more than two years, and we had saved up enough deposit money that the bank could not say no to us.

Now we had a house – and a mortgage! And these presented their own challenges. My God! I still vividly remember the first day our mortgage repayment came out. Being naïve about the whole thing, I was so depressed seeing that such a huge portion of our hard-earned money went to the bank as interest, with only a small amount going towards the principle. Anyway, we now had the gym, the mortgage, and we were planning a family. So, we decided to get married.

The challenges kept piling up. In 2015 we had a slightly bigger gym than the one we had in 2013 (60 square metres bigger to be exact), a house, we were married, and we welcomed into the world our beautiful son Malachi Wongueoh Nyenuh – who at the writing of this paragraph is four years old this morning. He was the light of our world. He was a dream come true. Nothing have I ever wanted more than being a dad, and he was a blessing.

But having a business to run, a mortgage, and a young family came with its own challenges. While it was okay to do 15-hour days without our son, now with him it was not okay. It was not what I had imagined or dreamed of. And definitely not something my wife could cope with this time. But this time business was not as it was in 2012, 2013, or even 2014, when I was doing those long hours because I wanted to. I now found myself doing those hours because unfortunately I *had* to. We had the overheads from the gym, the mortgage, and a family to provide for. As already mentioned in this book, being a personal trainer, I was trading my time for money. And because the money I made from trading my time paid the bills, I could not afford to be at home with my family as much as I wanted to or else the business would collapse, and we probably would lose our home.

And this created its own set of problems. I was tired and stressed from working long hours, and not being at home with my young family as much as I wanted to had me frustrated and easily irritated. My wife also felt tired, stressed, and – worst of all – alone. She missed me, she missed her family, and I missed her a lot. There were nights when I arrived home and she would be in tears. With getting used to and adjusting to being new parents, we struggled through what should have been the happiest time of our lives.

So, why am I sharing this story? I am sharing this story to highlight the dangers of running the rat race. A life that has no balance or satisfaction. Sometimes you have to take a step back and look at your life and ask yourself the hard questions: is this the kind of life I want to live? What is more important to me in my life? What is my purpose on this earth? Am I living out my own script or the script that was handed to me by my parents, society, or others?

The last question is important, because I found that even though I was not born in the western world, part of the reason why I found myself and my family in the situation that we did was because I was trying to live out the script handed to me by the western world, which is totally contrary to what I grew up in. A script that basically goes like this: 'You meet a girl; you buy a house; then you get married and have a family.' No doubt I wanted to have a family, but buying a house definitely did not need to be a priority.

But buying a house is celebrated by our society and western culture. If you buy a house, you are important, you are seen as a responsible person, and you are celebrated. I remember when we bought our house, we even got a mention in the newspaper. But what if it did not have to be that way? By no means am I saying buying property is a bad thing, because I understand property is one way that people create wealth for themselves and their families. But if you are not doing it from the script you have written for yourself, but out of the one that was handed to you by your society and culture, then it is also one way that people get themselves into a lot of debt and stress, which leads to no life/work balance. You end up working not because you want to or because you enjoy the work you do but because you have to, and most times that can suck the joy out of what you do and ultimately out of life. It did for me, but I found a way. I crawled out of the hole I had dug for myself by going back to living out the life that I wanted to live. By asking myself, what is more important? And what is my purpose on this earth? And, How Bad Do I Want It?

LIVING OUT SCRIPTS THAT ARE NOT OUR OWN

We all come into this world knowing nothing. Everything we know and do, we learned first from our parents, family and friends, society and culture, so if we grew up in a household where our parents did things a certain way, we tended to follow their example consciously or subconsciously, because our parents are our number one teacher. We follow the examples of our friends because we are social beings, and we will do everything in our power to try to fit in more times than not. We follow the trends of our society. If something is in trend, we try to fit in because not being a part will mean we are left behind, not cool, or out of touch. If our culture places value on certain things – good or bad – we blindly follow without investigating whether it is the right path for us.

Below are some scripts we live out, sometimes without questioning whether or not they are the right ones for us.

Parental scripts

If you grew up in a household where your parents set good examples for you to follows you will have a higher chance of following in their footsteps. I see a lot of people living out the scripts that were handed to them. And some of those scripts are not to their benefit. There are a lot of broken marriages as a result of these scripts, a lack of job satisfaction, and much unhappiness. If you grew up watching your parents fight all the time, you might think that is the norm; if they drank alcohol and smoked or ate junk food and fed you the same, your chances of following in that direction are higher. On the other hand, if they taught you good manners, how to be kind and polite, and to be content with what you have and live with integrity, you are more likely to adopt those values.

Let us consider this example: we have adults today who feel the need to have the biggest and finest houses, the flashiest and most expensive cars, jet-skis, boats, fancy gadgets – you name it. And I must say, it is totally okay to have all of these things as long as you are not burying yourself deeply in debt just to acquire them.

Unfortunately, that is not the case for a lot of people today. They put themselves into a lot of debt just to have the aforementioned items. So! What roles have parents got to play in this? Well, because I was not born here, and being a parent, I have been able to carefully study some aspects of the western culture and observe how it translates into our actions. Here is the role that parents play. In the western world when children are little, parents, especially grandparents, families, and even friends and acquaintances spoil them with countless gifts. Every birthday, Easter, Christmas. Children are spoilt with ridiculous numbers of presents.

Parents usually do this out of love and out of their own scripting that they received from their parents. They want their children to know they love them, and sometimes they feel the way they can express this love is by buying them numerous gifts. I get it. But there is also an underlying message and scripting that we give to children when we do this. We send them a message that one toy is not enough. Two toys are not enough. Three, four, five, or even six or ten presents are not enough. We help create this void where they keep wanting and expecting more.

I do not usually buy my son Malachi presents, and it is not because I do not love him. I show my love for him in other ways. And before you say 'poor kid', trust me – he gets spoilt with presents from his mother and grandparents. Just before his fourth birthday, after receiving the first three of his presents for Easter, my son said, 'Is that all I get?' I was mortified. We can try to justify this by saying they are just kids and that is what kids do, but that is not true. Kids do what we teach them. They learn what we tell them is right or wrong. These kids grow up into adults and end up getting in debt to collect things. Things that later end up in landfill. Australia as a nation per capita has more storage facilities and collects more waste at our dumpsites than most countries in the world. These children grow up to find themselves in a rat race where they have no time for themselves because they have to work to pay for their expensive lifestyle. What scripts are you writing for your children?

Social scripts

These are the social habits we live out to try to fit in with our friends, society, and trends or fads. We see our friends do something, and we try to do it too out of fear – fear of missing out, or FOMO as it is commonly referred to by hipsters. If our friends buy a nice car, a big house, or the latest phone or even a piece of jewellery, we want to do the same. It's keeping up with the Joneses. And that is primarily because we are social beings; we'd rather fit in because it's easier than trying not to. I remember sitting in a gathering with a group of friends where they were smoking marijuana and it was being passed around. When the lit weed came to me, I held it to my mouth and pretended to smoke it, just to fit in. If you have to do that, you are in the wrong social gathering. I did not reject weed because I was a saint. I did not smoke because of my prior scripting, which had a profound effect on me. I grew up in Africa. Unlike Australia, and most of the western world, we did not have mental health facilities for people who suffered from mental illnesses. As a kid, I saw many 'crazy people', as we called them in Africa, on the streets, eating out of dumpsites, wearing dirty clothes for days, and living on the streets. I was told from an early age that those people were like that because they smoked weed and did drugs, and that if I did not want to end up like one of them, I should avoid weed and drugs at all costs. That scripting had a powerful effect on my life.

Growing up in poverty and refugee camps, I really had nothing. When I moved to Australia, in my early days I would shop at the op shops and Target. When I started working and earning more money than I had ever seen before, I started to emulate the examples of what I saw to be cool. I learned that none of the people I hung around were shopping from those places that I shopped. So, I started buying nice things and being materialistic just to fit in.

This is sometimes no different in business. We want to keep up with what others are doing in our industry. We see our competitors do something and we want to try to match or do it better than them – we do not stop to think whether or not what they are doing is in line with *our* purpose or mission. Say, for example, a competitor moves to a bigger facility or opens up another facility; we try to copy them without even thinking about what their financial situation might be.

Here are two things I always remember when feeling this way, because being human means it's impossible to stop myself from having those thoughts of trying to keep up:

1. **Stay in your lane and play your own game.** Identify what your lane is and what your game is. Other people's lane and game could be completely different to mine.

2. **Not everything that glitters is gold.** I do not know what they are sacrificing to do what they are doing. It could be precious time. It is particularly important to remember what our mission or purpose is, because if we do not, that is when we start following the bright shiny objects – trying to do anything and everything because we see someone else do it. What is your mission and purpose?

Cultural scripts

Culture is defined as the characteristics and knowledge of a particular group of people, encompassing language, religion, cuisine, social habits, music, and arts. Generally, these are the scripts we are born into or develop along the way. For example, if you are born in a country that is predominantly Muslim, Christian, or Buddhist, you are likely to end up being one of those based on where you are born. If you are born in a country where the culture associates drinking alcohol with social gathering, your chances of picking up that script are high.

Cultural scripts have a huge influence on us. When our culture places value on certain behaviours and habits, it is regarded as the norm and can be extremely hard to break away from. For example: the vicious cycle of parents feeding their children sugary foods and drinks thinking they are showing them love; the idea that every social gathering should be celebrated with alcohol and junk food; or the idea that you need to buy a house before you get married, then you have a family.

There are no doubts that there are some very positive aspects to our cultural scripts, but my point is not to demonise or celebrate any habits of the scripts but to highlight the consequences of how blindly following a script that is not your own can lead to a life of no time. A life of dissatisfaction. A life where you do not really prioritise the important things in your life. A life where you do not live out the scripts that are in line with *your* purpose and meaning. I have been there, and I know what it feels like not only to be time poor but to be time poor because you do not have a choice due to your own prior choices. Whose script are you living?

NOT PUTTING IMPORTANT THINGS FIRST

Another reason I have found for why people are so time poor is that they do not put the important things first. And maybe part of that is because they have not quite worked out what the important things are in their lives. And that is why it's especially important to first sit down and ask yourself, if you have not already, what is the most important thing in my life? What would make the biggest difference in my personal and professional life if I were to do those things now? Why am I not doing them? If I could, what would I do? As Stephen Covey would say, we are too busy climbing up the ladder – we have not really made time to stop and check whether the ladder is leaning up against the right wall. It could be the ladder of success, fame, or wealth, but when that ladder is not in line with our purpose and mission in life it is all but a waste of time and ultimately life – doing things that are not really important.

When I started my business I had all the right intentions, but then I drifted towards living a scripted life. A script that was not my own. This shifted my ladder from the right wall to the wrong wall. So, I had to climb down from my ladder and move it to the wall that was most important to me: my family. Making time for my wife and two young children.

The problem I see with our busy society today is that we are busy chasing the wrong things. We do things because we see other people do them. We respond to urgent matters sometimes without realising that just because something is urgent does not mean it is important. We rarely make time for the important things. Things that benefit us in the long run. Things that when we do them, they help to make our lives and the lives of those around us better. A lot of people are doing what they have to do, not what they want to do. If you find yourself in this situation, I believe it is time you sit down and answer these questions:

- What is most important in my life?

- What is my life's purpose and meaning?

- What wall is my ladder leaning against?

The true answers to these questions will help change your life dramatically. If not immediately, eventually. But you have to commit to working on achieving what is more important to you. Because anything is possible if you want it bad enough.

NOW IS THE TIME FOR CHANGE

Change can be a scary thing, but it does not have to be, especially if it is one that improves your life and the lives of those around you. Here are four things to consider when embarking on the journey of change:

1. **Pleasure and pain:** We all seek two things in life. We are either trying to gain pleasure or avoid pain. All our decisions are based on these two principles. We make decisions because we want to gain pleasure, avoid pain, or both. I believe for a true change to occur, the pain of staying the same has to be far greater than the fear of the unknown or the pleasure we hope to achieve. For example, as previously mentioned in this book, when I made the decision to expand my gym from a 155-square-metre

gym with only 62 members to a 326-square-metre gym with huge overheads and the possibility of failing, it was purely out of pain. I was avoiding the pain of not seeing my wife enough. I was avoiding the pain of not seeing my son enough, and out of the painful realisation that if I had continued in that direction, I would not see him once he started going to school except on weekends. It was also out of the pain of working all those hours and then running the business at a loss. And not having anything to show for all the hard work. It was out of the pain of realising that this is not how I imagined running my own business would be.

There was no pleasure if I had stayed doing the same thing. Only pain I could see. This was the driver behind my decision. I was avoiding pain and hoping for pleasure. The pleasure of being able to spend more time with my wife and children, and to actually be there for them like I had envisaged. The pleasure of showing up to work happy to do what I do and not being stressed about how I was going to pay the bills. The pleasure of reaping the fruit of my labour. The pleasure of being able to run a business that was bigger than myself – a business that contributed to my local community as well as on a national and international scale. Fortunately, at the writing of this book, that decision has paid off, and we are now not only in a good place but heading in the right direction. We went from 62 members to now over 1000 members within the space of three years, and we are still growing and scaling. I now spend more time with my wife and children. I now spend more time working in a role that is most beneficial to my business and we are reaping the rewards. We do way more community charitable events now than we have ever been able to do before. We have a Muscle Garden Family that values what we are about.

My advice for making a meaningful and lasting change would be to first consider: what are you avoiding or seeking? Does the pain of staying the same outweigh the pain of making a change? Only when you can really quantify the depth of what is at stake can you achieve the level of success you are after.

2. **Personal bias:** Beware of personal bias when making changes. Personal bias is when we think we are better than we actually are. For example, it is the reason I think I am a better driver than my wife. Be realistic with yourself. I'm not saying talk yourself down, but be true to yourself. Know what you are really good at and the things that you are not so good at. Do not just blindly think that you are good at this or that without really taking the time to examine things. One common example I see all the time is when clients come in and do a fitness assessment and then realise that they are really not as fit as they initially thought they were. And those who put themselves down realise that they are not as bad as they thought they were. Make the time to check your personal bias.

3. **Confirmation bias:** Confirmation bias is looking for information and ideas to support your existing way of thinking. Or only looking for the things you want to hear. If you only accept the things you want to hear and reject the ones you do not, change will be difficult, and you will not grow as a person. Do not be afraid to challenge your way of thinking. We are all conditioned to see the world not as it is but as we are. If you only see the world from your point of view and your conditioning and only look for information to support your ideas and way of thinking, then you will only see the world from a limited perspective. Make time to challenge yourself and your thought processes. Challenge what you know and believe to be true. Look at things from various points of view and then make informed decisions.

Also, listen to the things that others say to you or about you. You learn through honest feedback. The best feedback is usually the hardest to give or receive. When I first moved to this country, one of the things I used to hear after I came out of my shell was that I was arrogant. Even my wife before we got together thought I was arrogant. This made me sit down to think about why people were calling me arrogant, when deep down in myself I did not think I was. One thing I learned early on in life was that if everyone thinks you have a problem, then maybe you have a problem. If you think everyone has a problem, then maybe you have a problem. So, I thought maybe I *am* arrogant. All these people cannot be wrong.

I sought to find out why I was perceived to be arrogant. And what I found was that people in Australia expressed themselves differently to how people did where I came from. I was confident, and I did not mind saying what was on my mind, and I did not mind talking about myself. This was not the Aussie way. People are more laidback and modest in the way they express themselves here. This realisation had a huge impact on my life. Since 2012, I cannot remember one single person saying to my face that I am arrogant. That is not to say that they are not thinking it, but I believe the way I express myself now is a lot better than it used to be. Pay attention to your critics. Not everyone who criticises you is a 'hater'. Some criticisms will help you grow.

4. **Opportunity cost:** This is defined as the loss of other alternatives when one alternative is chosen. If time is the most valuable currency in the world then every second spent is an opportunity that is far too great to be wasted. We can always earn more money, but time we cannot. The time you spend doing one thing is an opportunity that you could spend doing another. So, ask yourself – what are you doing with your time that could be far more important or valuable if you did something else? Say, for example, the time spent watching TV is at the cost of the time that could be spent reading a book, writing an article, making someone's day, or volunteering at a

local charitable shop or organisation. The time spent on aimless chatter is at the cost of the time that could be invested in deep, meaningful work or time with your partner or children. What could you do with the time you spend scrolling through your social media feeds? Think about that.

What are you spending your time doing, and what is it costing you? Remember this quotation in everything that you do:

'The cost of a thing is the amount of "life" we must exchange for it.' – Henry David Thoreau

Let's look at the two types of change processes that people often take. They are 'unintentional change' and 'intentional change':

1. **Unintentional change** – starts with:

   - *Denial:* In this stage there is a problem, but you refuse to recognise it or accept that it is a problem. For example, an overweight person may think they are fine as long as they are moving around and going about their daily activities. They may not really want to accept or acknowledge that being overweight is a problem that poses many health risks and it is one that needs their attention. At this stage they are in denial.

   - *Judgement:* At this stage they go from being in denial to recognising that there is a problem, but the step they take is that they start judging themselves in comparison to others. They engage in negative self-talk. They think they are not good enough. They get awfully hard on themselves.

   - *Control:* In this stage the person goes from judging themselves to trying to control the situation. They want to stop their bad habit, so they start to put in measures to try to control it. And usually how they do this is by telling themselves that, 'I would only do this if I do this other habit'. That other habit is usually not a good habit either. For example, a smoker would say, 'I want to control the number of cigarettes I smoke per week, so what I will do is, I will only have a cigarette when I have a drink'. The problem with this is that usually what happens is you notice the amount of time they drink goes up. So, not only are they smoking, they are also now drinking with smoking.

- *Reaction:* At this stage we start to react. We are not proactive but reactive to the change process and the decisions we make. For example, an overweight person may decide to join a gym without any strategy or plan in place. They join the gym for a couple of months, and when they do not see the results they are looking for immediately, they quit. A smoker may wake up one day and decide, *that is it, I am quitting.* Only to find themselves back at it again after a short while.

- *No positive action:* At this stage, the person sort of gives up. Nothing anyone can say to them that will make them change their mind. Every action they take is not in their best interests for change. At this point you hear family and friends say, 'We have tried everything'. Despite their best efforts, this person does not take any positive action. The person even gets to thinking that they have tried everything, and nothing works.

2. **Intentional change** – on the other hand – starts with:

- *Awareness:* The first step to change is awareness. Being aware or recognising that there is a problem is imperative to your success in changing any problem. It is better than denying there is a problem. Awareness is being honest with yourself and saying, 'I have a problem and I am going to do something about it'.

- *Acknowledgement:* Is accepting that you have a problem, but this time instead of judging yourself, you acknowledge it without any negative self-talk or comparisons to others. You identify the consequences of this problem and how it is impacting your life and the lives of your loved ones.

- *Choice:* Unlike trying to control the situation or problem, you must realise you have a choice to make a change or stay the same. Instead of doing it impulsively, you realise that you have the ability to choose your response in any given situation in life. Someone can have a gun to your head and you still have a choice. As Viktor Frankl said, our freedom to choose is the last of our human freedoms that no one can take away. It is an immensely powerful thing to have – choice. Made correctly and our lives can be made better, but when the wrong choices are made, life can be miserable. Once you connect to the source of what is most important in your life, your choices become somewhat easier. You put the important things first. You choose to exercise because it improves your physical being; you choose to spend time with your spouse and kids because it enriches your relationship with them; you choose good habits that serve you for good in the long run over habits that give you instant gratification but long-term pain. You have the power and privilege to choose to do the things that carry the most weight on the 'importance scale'. And by doing this, you get to live a balanced life that is full of meaning.

- *Strategy:* You then devise a plan of action for how you are going to implement and execute your choice. You put this action plan in place to follow. Your plan must factor in your 'why' and what, how, and when you are going to execute it. For example, an overweight person who decides to do something about their health and weight by going to the gym and making healthy choices about what they eat may have this strategy. They may decide to start exercising because they want to improve their health. They choose to exercise at least three times per week – every Monday, Wednesday, and Friday for 45 minutes between the hours of 6am and 7am. They may choose to get a fitness assessment done to see where they are starting from, as well as getting a gym program to follow. And they may also get a meal plan to follow and have someone to hold them accountable.

- *Action and measurement:* You then start to measure and track every action. What is measured is managed and, most importantly, improved. Using our example above, the overweight person may decide to do weekly weigh-ins to see their progress. And since the scales do not tell the full story of what is going on in their body, they may also choose to do a body scan every four to six weeks to see their progress. They may keep a journal documenting their progress. They may also keep track of how many days per week they are going to the gym, and how many weeks they have been consistent. They may have an accountability partner or group to keep them accountable to their goals and hold them to a high standard.

TIME: THE MOST VALUABLE CURRENCY

When the Global Financial Crisis hit in 2008, so many people lost *a lot* of money. Many economies around the world went broke. People lost their jobs, houses, and cars. In my mining town of Mackay, when the mining downturn hit in 2012, for a few years, life was tough. Lots of people lost their jobs, and I saw many businesses close down around me. I even had clients who had to stop their personal training because, quite simply, if you cannot afford to put food on the table for your family, the last thing you want to be doing is paying for personal training sessions.

I ran my business at a loss for two years in a row. As bad as things were, it was a moment in time. And though there are still some people picking up the pieces from the damage caused by the Global Financial Crisis and mining downturn, some of those countries that went broke have now managed to get their economies back on track. Lots of people have been able to get their lives back on track; some have regained the money they lost and even made more money than they previously had. Jobs have been restored, houses bought again, new business ventures opened. Personally, in my case we were fortunate enough to go from being broke to being profitable. My point is, when you lose money you can get it back, but when you lose time, it is impossible to get it back. And that's why it is important how we choose to spend our time on this earth and the people or things we spend this time with. Do not get too caught up chasing money that you forget to make time for the things that truly matter in life. I hear stories all the time of millionaires who would give up their wealth if it meant they could go back in time to be there for their children when they were growing up. Millionaires who wish they had paid more attention to their marriage, their family, their health, and would pay any amount of money to go back in time and change things. And even people who are not millionaires but those chasing wealth, fame, and social status or job positions.

Success can come at a terrible cost; money can make life easy, but it is not everything in life. Often the best things in life do not even cost money. A simple life is sometimes better than a rich life that is full of regrets. Now is the time to change and to refocus where, how, and what you spend your time on. It could be the difference between a life of regrets and one full of peace, meaning, and fulfilment.

TIME TO SAY *NO*

Success is not determined by the quality of things you say 'yes' to but by the quality of things you say 'no' to. Warren Buffett is known for saying: 'The difference between successful people and really successful people is that really successful people say no to almost everything.' Being human beings, the initial instinct for most of us is to please other human beings. We want to gain favour. We want them to like us and be happy with us. And sometimes, we will bend over backwards to do this. We will take the shirt off our back and give to another person. We will give up our time for other people, even if it is time that we really need to spend on ourselves, family, or an important project that needs completing.

We do all this because sometimes we genuinely care and want to help, and other times sadly because we do not have a bigger 'yes' inside of us, so it is hard to say 'no'. Most of the time it's because we want to avoid friction. It is easier to say 'yes' than it is to say 'no'. We think that by saying 'no' we are being mean, selfish, and not kind. We fear that by saying 'no' we will offend people.

But what is saying 'yes' all the time costing you? I do not mean to sound selfish here, but what could you have done with the time that you spent trying to please someone? And how much difference would that time have made to your life, family, and work? Was it in line with your purpose? What did it cost you? Have you ever done something for someone and then later regretted doing it? How many times has that happened? When you have a clear answer to these questions, you realise that you do not need to say yes just for the sake of it. When our life is in order, when we have control over the things that are important in our life, we can choose the things we say 'yes' or 'no' to. We can say 'yes' to the things that are important to us, the ones that are in line with our purpose, mission, or drive in life, and say 'no' to the ones that are not. It is easy to say 'no' when we have a bigger 'yes' burning inside of us.

When you say 'yes' to someone or something, you are not just saying 'yes' to that person or thing. You are also saying 'no' to yourself and the things that you could have done.

Steve Jobs once said: 'If you want to make everyone happy, don't be a leader – sell ice cream.' You may think, 'But I am not a leader of a company or anything of the sort,' but you *are* the leader of your life. And maybe the leader of your household, or your young children. The decisions you make affect not only your life but the lives of those around you. Your loved ones. Carefully choose the things you say 'yes' to and do not be afraid to say 'no'. Do not seek to please everyone to your own detriment.

And it may not just be saying 'no' to other people or situations; it could be you saying 'no' to yourself. Saying 'no' to habits that do not benefit you long term, saying 'no' to self-sabotaging beliefs and habits. Saying 'no' to negative associations and gatherings that do not benefit you or that are not in line with your purpose.

Say 'no'. Have a bigger 'yes' inside.

Remember this: you cannot pour from an empty cup.

TIME TO LOCK IN THE RIGHT MINDSET

Our mind controls everything we do in life. If the base from which our actions flow is flawed, our actions will also be flawed. The things you tell yourself and your beliefs could sometimes be holding you back. So be mindful of the stories you tell yourself. They could propel you forward in life or hold you back.

Develop a growth mindset. Regardless of what you have been telling yourself or have been told, you can do anything if you put your mind to it. If you want it bad enough. It is the only reason why a refugee kid like myself, hopeless and helpless as they come, can move to this country and achieve the things I have today. Which, to some people, is not really much, but when you come from where I come from and experience the situations that I have been through, you will appreciate that what I have achieved is huge.

It is never where you are right now in your life that matters but where you want to be and how bad you really want to get there. I wake up every day and tell myself that I know where I come from. I was born in a country that went through 14 years of civil war. Millions of people died, including close family. I know the continent I left behind. People are suffering and dying every day. Many have no jobs – living in hardship and poverty. I was blessed to make it out. My time here will not be taken for granted. There are millions of people in Africa who wish they were in my position today or had the opportunity and privilege that I have to be living in Australia today. I will not waste my time.

Lock in the right mindset. The mindset to be better than you are today. Seek continuous growth and improvement. Look for areas in your life that you can improve on. And recognise the areas that you are doing well in. Dare to do something bigger than yourself. Something meaningful. Set aside time to check in with yourself and examine your thoughts. Socrates once said, 'Know thyself', and, 'The unexamined life is not worth living'.

TIME TO REALLY INTERPRET YOUR GOALS

Understand what a goal is. Understand what it is that you really want. Your deepest, inner-most desire, and be crystal clear on why you want it. Set aside time to write down your goals and, more importantly, write down your action plan. The strategy that you are going to use to achieve your goals. Identify the resources needed – people, organisations, equipment, knowledge that you are going to have to gain to achieve each goal.

Let us consider this example: I always had it in the back of my mind that one day I will write a book. But I had never written a book before. I did not even have a clue on where and how to start. So, I did some research. I took up a one-year business course and, as part of that course, I learned the framework for how to write a book.

Some goals are going to require you to stretch yourself and get outside of your comfort zone. The real trick then is not to chase the goal but to become the person who can achieve that goal. To embrace and fall in love with the process and enjoy the journey. I did not become an author the day my book was published; I was an author when I started writing my book. Another example: I went into business with pure passion. I had a love for helping people and

I had a passion for health and fitness. I saw the way my industry was run, and I believed it could be done better, so I started my own business. Passion and love alone can only get you so far. As my business grew, I set goals to learn more about business. To become a better businessman, to learn to take a step back and focus on the vital things and let others do more of the functional work – the day-to-day running of the business. To learn how to be a better leader, employer, how to grow the business and turn it into a business that does good.

Track and keep a written record of your progress. What areas are you doing well in and what other areas could you improve on? Set aside time to think about your goals. How is one goal going to change your life and the lives of those around you? Who are you going to become as a result of that goal, and what impact will you make as a result of becoming that person? If you want something bad enough, be willing to become the person who is capable of achieving that goal.

TIME TO VOW TO HAVE GOOD NUTRITION

The majority of us started our nutrition journey on the wrong foot. As kids our parents fed us whatever they thought or knew was right. It is not their fault. Most of them did not even know the difference between what was healthy and what was not, and even if they knew, they were too powerless to do something about it because, like you, their own parents fed them in the same manner that they fed you. But now you are a grown-up. You are educated, you live in the information age, and you know the difference between what is healthy and what is not, or at least you have read in this book how to get help. Now, vow to have good nutrition. You have the power and you owe it yourself, to your loved ones, and to your moods and how you feel. Make a vow that you will eat the food that is good for your health and that you will feed your children, if any, the same way. The Bible says in the book of Proverbs Chapter 22 Verse 6: 'Train up a child in the way he should go: and when he is old, he will not depart from it.'

The decisions you make and the actions you take affect not only your life but the lives of those around you also. The food you put in your mouth has the power to sustain life or take it away. It has the power to boost your energy level or drain it. The food you consume has the power to improve your health or make you ill. Food is medicine. If you want to improve the quality of your life, start by paying attention to what you put into your mouth. Make a vow to yourself. Vow to have food that nourishes your body and improves your overall wellbeing. Food that sustains you. Now is the time to make that vow. Your body will thank you for it.

TIME TO INCLUDE EXERCISE

One of the biggest excuses people give today for not exercising is a lack of time. And honestly, some people are genuinely time poor. But as we talked about earlier in this step, one of the reasons they are time poor is because they are spending way too much time on urgent things and not important things. They are too busy climbing the proverbial ladder of success and have not really stopped to check whether the ladder is leaning against the right wall. They are living out scripts that were handed to them by their parents, society, or culture, and have not really stopped to figure out what their own script is; what is it that is really more important to them?

From what I know and what mountains of research suggests, exercise is one of those things that we cannot afford to *not* make time for. Not making time for exercise is essentially making time for a sub-optimum life. A life of low energy levels, illnesses and diseases, weak bones and muscles, foggy head, and the list goes on. No matter how busy your life is, it is time to include exercise.

Do not find time to exercise, *make* time to exercise. Plan your days, and more importantly your weeks. Pick out days and times out of the week when you are going to exercise. Plan your workouts. I am not saying that it's going to be easy at first; no, it will not be. I am not saying that you are going to see results right away; no, you will not. But what I am saying is, do it anyway. It will be worth it. You will get better.

A common example could be, 'I am going to exercise three times per week on every Monday, Wednesday and Friday'. And then pick a time that you are going to exercise. If you are not a morning person, do not pick morning time slots. Way too much friction, and the more friction, the less likely you will do it. Pick the afternoon if that is what works best for you. If you do not trust yourself that after work you are going to exercise then stick to the morning. Get it over and done with and carry on with your day. But above all, include exercise in your life, in your days, in your weeks. Put it in your diary and stick to it.

You might not be perfect at first, but the plan is first writing it in and then starting small. Your first few weeks might only be 30-minute workouts, and even if it is less than that, that's fine. The idea is to get into the routine of showing up. Fall in love with the process first, then you can build up from there. If you start too hard too early, chances are you will not last.

Include exercise in your life.

TIME TO NAIL YOUR HABITS

Habits – good or bad – shape who you are. They sometimes represent how people refer to you. Say, for example, if you have a bad habit of drinking alcohol and getting drunk often, people might call you an alcoholic or a drunkard. If you have a good habit of exercising and eating healthily, people might identify you with being fit and healthy. It is time to nail your habits, and the important thing to remember is the habits you want to nail are the ones that will benefit you in the long run. The ones that are in line with your purpose and meaning in life. The ones you want people to remember you by. Some examples could be making more time for your family and loved ones, being a good human being, being kind and loving, making time to exercise and making healthy food choices, making time to read, meditate, or write, and doing what's right even when there is no one around. That is integrity. It is a principle and value to live by and it is a habit worth practising.

As the saying goes, big things come in little packages, and good habits are no different. Habits start small and they compound over time. Nailing your habits will take time. There are no quick fixes, fads, or trends that will help, so do not expect it to be easy. In my profession, I see people chasing quick fixes, fads, and trends all the time, and some of those are for fast weight loss – they want results like yesterday. But the reality is nothing that is worth having in life comes easily. Important things in life usually take time to achieve, and they sometimes last a lifetime when the habits that achieved them are maintained. There is nothing quick fix about developing a good habit.

Nailing your habits will sometimes require you to dig deeper within yourself to find out not only why each habit is important to you and why they are even worth nailing in the first place, but also to tap into some internal motivation. To ask yourself – who am I? What am I capable of? What are the things I have achieved in my life before, and what are they compared to this new habit that I am trying to form? I had to do that when deciding to limit the time I spent on my phone. I realised I was the kind of person who was disciplined enough to quit drinking alcohol and exercise at least five times per week. Why then could I not limit the time I spent on my phone? I found out that I could. But only after I tapped into my soul and found the deep meaning and motivation. Less time on my phone meant disconnecting from people who were far away – most of whom I did not even know – and connecting with those who were close, like my wife and kids. Within the first few weeks of cutting down my screen time, I looked at the stats on my phone. I got my weekly emails from Facebook telling me how my page had performed, and all the numbers were down, but it was okay. I still had a business that was doing great. The time I lost being on my phone or social media, I gained in connecting with my wife and children. Extra time with them is always more important. And whenever

I am slipping, I can always count on my wife, my accountability partner, to remind me of what is more important.

If the habits you are trying to nail are not deeply anchored to a source that is far greater and more meaningful than not nailing the habits, chances are you will not be successful. It is time to nail your habits – the ones that are most important to you.

TIME TO MAKE TIME FOR THE THINGS THAT ARE MOST IMPORTANT

What are the most important things in your life? This is a crucial question. Before you even start thinking about making time for the most important things in your life, you must first know what those things are. So, if you have not really thought about or known what those things are, now might be a good time to do so. Take some time to think about those things. What are they and why are they the most important things in your life? If you were to make time for those things, what are you losing and what are you gaining in return?

Individually, we all have different things that are important to us on different levels. For example, what I personally find important may not be the same for you, but being humans, we all have some things in common. And due to these commonalities, there are some universal things that when we all pay attention to them and spend time on them, we can live a life full of balance, meaning, and contribution. They include improving our physical being, our spiritual being, our minds, and our social interactions with other human beings. It's important that we make time to satisfy these four dimensions of our being.

Making time for the most important things in your life will not be easy. In fact, it will require you to reposition your values. As Jordan B. Peterson said in his book *12 Rules for Life: An antidote to chaos*:

Sometimes when things are not going well it's not the world that is the cause. The cause is instead that which is currently most valued subjectively and personally. Why? Because the world is revealed to an indeterminate degree through the template of your values. If the world you are seeing is not the world you want, therefore, it is time to examine your values. It is time to rid yourself of your current presuppositions. It is time to let go. It might even be time to sacrifice what you love best so that you can become who you might become instead of staying who you are.

TIME TO LOOK IN THE MIRROR

When there is no one else around and you look in the mirror, who do you see? Change or personal improvement – like improving your fitness – is not about being better than another person. It is about being better than the person you were yesterday in line with your current values or who you want to become. So, when you look in the mirror, you are looking at your only competition. You are looking at the most important project you will ever work on, and trust me, though it may not be easy, the results will be more than worth it.

It is not where you are in your life right now that matters. It is where you want to be and how bad you really want to get there. And the decisions you make today will help you get there and ultimately determine the story you tell tomorrow. Yesterday is gone, so start today, because tomorrow is a day that never comes. I often hear people say: 'One day I will start exercising. One day I will do this and that.' The reality is, there are seven days in a week and 'one day' is not one of them – so start *now*. Start today! If you want it bad enough, nothing is impossible.

How Bad Do You Want It?

CONCLUSION

What is your best life? In this book you've just read, I've outlined what I believe to be a framework to living your best life. But I do understand that education is often given from the point of view and conditioning of the educator. With this in mind, I am aware that your definition of living your best life may be totally different to what I have written and elaborated on in this book. If that is the case, I urge you to explore that. Find out for yourself what it means to live your best life. What would you need? What are the pieces that would need to fall into place for you to know you are living your best life? And what would you need to do to make that happen? I wholeheartedly encourage you to do that.

But if you believe this framework, though I lay no claim to it being exhaustive, will help you live your best life, then I urge you to apply it. Knowledge is only potential power. Applied knowledge is true power. Apply the things you've read in this book. You won't be perfect. Though I wrote them, I myself am not perfect. The goal is to keep trying over and over again and over time, some things will become easier. Like:

Mindset – you will get better at knowing if your mindset about situations in life is the right one or not. You'll be mindful of the stories you tell yourself. Because you now understand that the stories you tell yourself have the power to shape who you are as a person. You'll question whether they are empowering or self-sabotaging beliefs.

Goals – you will take the time to really get clear on what it is that you want and why you want it. If your why is big enough and if it ties in with who you are as a person and the things you value, you will find a way to make that possible. You'll look for people, resources and whatever you need to do to achieve that goal because where there is a will, there is always a way.

Nutrition – armed with the understanding that food can be both beneficial and detrimental to your health, you will learn to question the things you put in your body. While food can be used for energy, sustenance, health and growth of our body, it can also have the opposite effect if we consume food for the wrong reasons or the wrong kinds of foods.

Exercise – with the understanding that our body is a garden of muscles and like a garden of plants, without proper care we will look undesirable and eventually wither away and die, you will look after your own garden of muscles because the benefits of physical activities far outweigh the effort it takes to keep active. Our quality of life basically depends on this one step. We were made to move.

Habits – our habits shape who we are. As Will Durant said, and I quote: 'We are what we repeatedly do.' Excellence, then, is not an act, but a habit. To achieve excellence (not perfection) we must repeatedly do and practice that which it is that we want to achieve excellence in. Like practicing all the steps in this book repeatedly and the habits that we want to define us.

Time – you will get better at making time for the things that are most important to you. Things that give you meaning and fulfillment. Time is truly the most valuable currency in this world and that is because time equals life. If we waste our time, we are wasting our life. Make time for what truly matters to you.

Finally, I've made some references in this book about stories from my life and I want to clarify:

- Leaving the mines to start a personal training business. In no way whatsoever, am I suggesting that you should leave the mines because I did. Living in a mining town, I understand how important mining is to our local and national economies. I also understand how many people have managed to provide a great life for their families while making the choice to be on mine sites week in, week out. My point was to explain that my personal definition of living my best life and the picture of the life I wanted to live would not have been possible had I stayed in the mines. And if this is you also, then my story was to paint the picture that anything, including leaving the mines to pursue your heart's desires, is possible if you want it bad enough.

- Not wanting my marriage to fall apart because I didn't want my son growing up in two separate homes and that it wasn't the life I envisaged when I thought of having a family. Please also allow me to say that by no means am I suggesting staying in a marriage for those reasons. Some marriages aren't safe to be in, including for children, if any. And in this case, if all else fails, it is sometimes better to be apart than together. The challenges I faced in my marriage weren't unique to just my family. And because they were things we could work through and because we wanted to be together more than we wanted to be apart and provide a safe environment for our children to be loved and nurtured, we made it work. We wanted it bad enough.

- I painted a picture that making time for my family was very important to me and that's because it is. But I do understand this may not be the case for everyone and I am not saying that it should be. So again, I want to say that what's important to me does not necessarily have to be what's important to you. But the point I want to make is find out what that is and make time for it, whatever it may be.

Throughout this book, you have read my story. I was a young kid who survived war, lived in refugee camps with no hope, and today I've arrived at this point in my life where I am living my best life. A life full of energy and vitality, to be able to do business and family life well. A life where I am in the best mental and physical shape of my life. A life of being a good role model to not only my children but to others in my community. And a life of contribution to causes that are dear to my heart.

What I want to say to you is that, Michael Jordan once said and I quote: 'I've never lost a game. I just ran out of time.' Friend, the good news is life is not a basketball game or a football, rugby, soccer or even a cricket game. You've still got time. Life is short, but not as short as many people make it out to be. You've still got time to have, be and do what you might have done because …

It is not where you are today in your life that matters, but where you want to be and how bad you really want to get there.

How Bad Do You Want It?

ACKNOWLEDGEMENTS

First and foremost, I want to give my heartfelt thanks and utmost gratitude to the creator of the universe, my God almighty for all of the blessings he has bestowed upon my life. I wouldn't be in the position I am in today if it wasn't for his help. All glory to you, Lord.

To my beautiful wife Jessica, thank you so much for all of your support and love. I may not give you all the credit you deserve as often as I should but thank you for sharing this life with me and for loving me. I couldn't think of a better person to do life with. Your caring and compassionate heart and the love you have for me and our children is unmeasurable. Thank you.

To my children Malachi, Rosa and Korrioh, thank you for enriching my life with the joy and happiness that you bring. I couldn't be any prouder to be your father. My greatest fantasy in life was to be a dad and you kids are my true legacy. It is my hope that you'll grow up valuing the meaning of hard work and going after what you want in life with relentless determination. It is my hope also that I can be the best dad you'll ever need.

To Denise, thank you so much for helping a total stranger from Africa come to Australia and live in your home to be able to live the life I live today. Totally mind blowing what you've done, and I thank

God for allowing our paths to cross. You are utterly amazing, and I believe the world needs more people like you. People who do not need much to do amazing things for others. Thank you for giving me this opportunity. I will forever be grateful.

To my mother Jessie, thank you for bringing me into this world and nurturing me with all the love I needed when I was just a child. Thank you for your endless prayers upon my life and for my family. Even when our paths were separated, you never ceased to pray for me. You've been through a lot in life and yet your heart for others is always for their best. Thank you.

Thank you to my Muscle Garden Family (personal training clients, gym members and all past and current staff) for believing and accepting what I started. Together, we have built something that is the envy of town. Muscle Garden would not be where it is today without you amazing people who have made it your gym of choice in a town where there isn't a shortage of gyms. Thank you!

Special thanks to Scot Alcorn, Stephen and Caryl Turpin, Chantel Woods, Rachel and Jordon Euler, Wayne James, Craig Stewart, Greg and Tanya Jasch, Andrew Dean and Deb Turvey, Mitchell Binney, Jeff and Donna Twomey, Peter Goodworth, Peter and Tammy Lando and more for the key roles you played in the expansion of our gyms right back from 2016 to where we are today. Thank you for investing your time as well as your money and other resources to get us to where we are today. There are many of you that I could name here, but I believe we would need another book just for that. Thank you, MG Fam! Let's keep striving to be better tomorrow than we are today.

Thank you to the team at Dent Global for providing the training platform that among other things has made this book possible. Also, a massive thank you to my accountability partners: Emily Hayles, Michael Back and Matt Davis for keeping me accountable to get this book out. Thank you, team, let's keep making our dent in the universe.

Also, a huge thank you to Michael Hanrahan Publishing for making this book a reality. Michael, Anna and the rest of the team, thank you for helping me every step of the way to get this book out.

Last but certainly not the least, a massive thank you to all those who accepted me wholeheartedly regardless of my background and wanted the best for me when I first moved to this country. Even to those who told me to "go back to where you came from" when I first moved here, thank you. You have all helped to shape me into the person I am today. So, thank you!

Thank you to the community of Mackay for your support and thank you Australia for being true to the fact that if anyone has a 'fair dinkum go' they can have, do and be anything they want in life. Thank you and God bless.

Kay in Africa

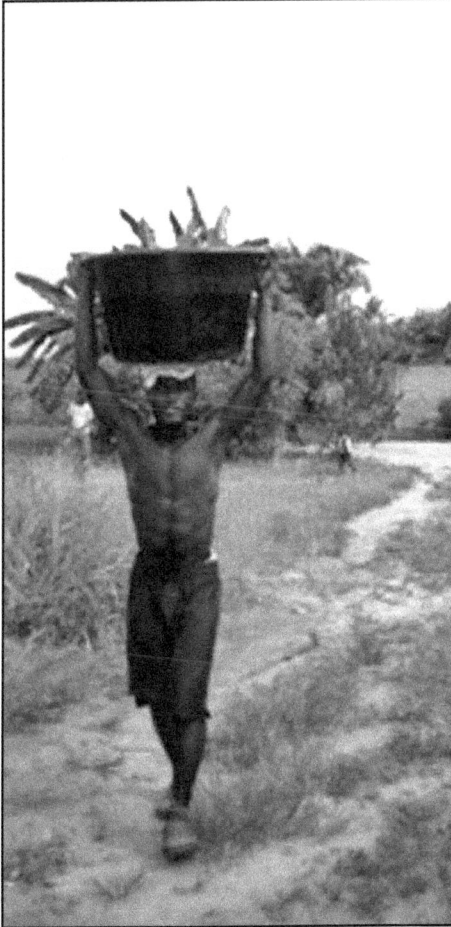
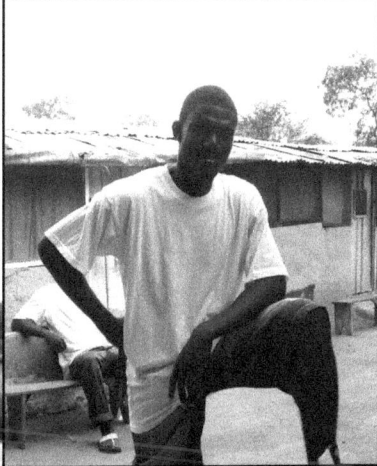
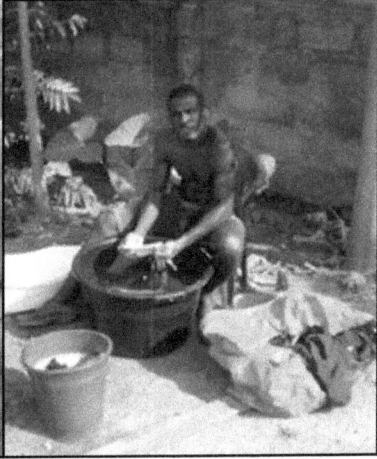

APPENDIX A
HEALTHY RECIPES

Rainbow Breakfast Bowl with Eggs and Avocado

|Serves 4|

8 fresh eggs

2 avocados

1 lemon

Salt and pepper

1 tablespoon garlic salt

2 capsicums, sliced thinly

4 carrots, sliced thinly

1 large brown onion, cut into small wedges

1 head of broccoli, chopped roughly

2 zucchinis, sliced thinly

1 cup of corn

1 cup of peas

1 sweet potato, peeled and grated

Olive oil

1 teaspoon chilli flakes

Method

1. Add olive oil to a pan over medium heat. Add all ingredients to the pan except the eggs and avocado and stir-fry until vegetables soften. Sit to the side.
2. While the vegetables are cooking, slice the two avocados in half, remove the seed and skin and sit to the side.
3. In a non-stick pan over medium heat, pan fry the eggs. For sunny side up eggs cook until the whites are set. For well-done eggs, turn the eggs to sunny side down.
4. Remove from the heat.
5. In a serving bowl add a serving of the rainbow vegetables. Top with 2 eggs and ½ avocado. Serve with a lemon wedge.
6. Eat and enjoy!

Acai Bowl with Seasonal Fruit and Grain-free Nut Granola

|Serves 4|

4 packets of frozen Amazonia Acai Pure
4 frozen bananas, sliced
1 frozen mango, diced
Sliced seasonal fruit
2 tablespoons grain-free nut granola (as per recipe on page 201)

Method

1. In a Vitamix or equivalent place the frozen acai, frozen banana and frozen mango.
2. Turn the Vitamix on to 1 and gradually increase to 10. Using the tamper, push the ingredients down to the blade until smooth and combined. This should take no longer than 60 seconds. Sit to the side.
3. In a bowl sprinkle a small amount of the grain-free nut granola. Spoon on frozen acai mixture. Cover with your choice of seasonal fruit toppings and sprinkle more grain-free nut granola on top.
4. Eat and enjoy!

Chia Pudding

|Serves 4|

¼ cup chia seeds
1 cup coconut milk
1 tablespoon honey
1 teaspoon vanilla extract
1 teaspoon ground cinnamon
Toppings: nuts, seeds, fruit

Method

1. Combine all ingredients in a small airtight container, glass jar or breakfast bowl.
2. Store in the fridge overnight.
3. Serve with your choice of toppings.

Banana Pancakes

|Serves 4|

3 ripe bananas, mashed
2 eggs
4 heaped tablespoons wholemeal flour
1 tablespoon cinnamon
Olive oil (or alternative)
Toppings: Drizzled honey, chopped almonds and sliced banana

Method

1. In a blender combine all ingredients and blend until smooth.
2. Heat a non-stick frying pan over medium heat. Grease pan with olive oil.
3. Pour mixture in pan and cook until bubbles appear on the surface. Turn and cook for a further minute.
4. Transfer to a plate and repeat with the remaining mixture.
5. Serve with a drizzle of honey, chopped almond and sliced banana.

Overnight Oats

|Serves 4|

2 cups rolled oats
1 apple, peeled and grated
1 tablespoon cinnamon
6 dates, chopped
½ cup raw almonds, chopped
1 tablespoon honey
2 cups soy milk (or alternative)
⅓ cup shredded coconut
Toppings: nuts, seeds, fruit

Method

1. Combine all ingredients in an airtight container.
2. Store in the fridge overnight.
3. Serve with your choice of toppings.

Baked Eggs

|Serves 4|

8 ripe large tomatos, diced
8 button mushrooms, chopped
½ brown onion
8 basil leaves
2 tablespoons garlic salt
4–6 eggs
Olive oil
1 tablespoon chilli flakes (optional)

Method

1. Heat olive oil in an ovenproof frying pan over medium heat.
2. Add onion and cook for 1 minute. Add mushroom and cook for a further minute.
3. Add diced tomatoes, garlic salt and chilli flakes (optional). Stir to combine and lower heat to low. Cook until tomatoes have softened, and it resembles chutney-like consistency. If your tomatoes are not juicy, you may need to add a small amount of water.
4. Crack eggs over tomatoes and cover the pan with a lid until eggs are cooked.
5. Serve and enjoy!

Grain-free Nut Granola

½ cup coconut flakes

2 cups slivered almonds

1 ¼ cup raw pecans

1 cup raw walnuts

3 tablespoons chia seeds

1 tablespoon ground cinnamon

2 tablespoons coconut oil

¼ cup pepitas

Pinch of salt

¼ cup honey

Method

1. Preheat oven to 160 degrees.
2. In a large mixing bowl combine the coconut, nuts, chia seeds, cinnamon and salt.
3. In a small saucepan over low heat, warm the coconut oil and honey until combined. Remove from the heat and pour over the dry ingredients.
4. Spread mixture evenly over a large baking tray sheet and bake for 20 minutes, stirring every 5 minutes. Cook until golden brown.
5. Remove from the heat and allow to cool completely before storing in an airtight container in the fridge.
6. Use as toppings for breakfast or as a snack. Enjoy!

Fusion Scrambled with Lime Avocado

|Serves 4|

1-inch ginger, chopped finely
1 tablespoon crushed garlic
2 birds eye chilli, chopped finely
½ brown onion, chopped finely
1 tablespoon butter (or alternative)
1 tablespoon mixed dry herbs
8–12 eggs
3 avocados
½ lime, juiced
Salt and pepper
Baby spinach

Method

1. In a medium sized bowl, add avocado and juice of lime and mash until combined. Season with salt and pepper and sit to the side.
2. In a pan over medium heat add butter, ginger, garlic, onion, chilli and dried herbs. Sauté until onion softens. Meanwhile, crack your eggs into a bowl and whisk them until bubbles form.
3. Pour eggs into the pan and allow to sit for 1–2 minutes until it begins to set. Using a spatula work your way around the outside of the eggs, pulling the sides into the middle. Keep doing this until there is a small amount of liquid remaining. Add the baby spinach and continue pulling the eggs to the middle until there is no more liquid remaining.
4. To serve, add equal portions of eggs to a bowl and top with avocado.
5. Eat and enjoy!

Butterfly Prawns with Quinoa Salad

|Serves 4|

1kg of raw prawns
¼ Kent pumpkin
2 garlic cloves, crushed
1 small handful of mint
1 tablespoon chilli flakes
Olive oil
Juice of 3 lemons
½ cup quinoa
¼ cup pepitas
1 teaspoon fennel seeds
Salt and pepper
1 teaspoon sumac
1 teaspoon coriander, ground
½ teaspoon cumin, ground
1 small handful of fresh coriander
¼ cup of roasted hazelnuts, crushed
1 red onion, cut into small wedges

Method

Prawn preparation

1. Remove the head of the prawns by either twisting off or using a sharp knife.
2. Using kitchen scissors, snip off the feelers and legs.
3. Starting from behind where the head was, cut the shell along the middle of the prawn's body all the way to the tail.
4. Using a sharp knife, make an incision through the prawn being careful not to cut through the shell.
5. Open the prawn up like a butterfly and press it down gently so that it stays that way. Remove the intestinal tract.

6. Place prawns in a large bowl with the juice of 2 lemons, 1 garlic clove crushed, 1 tablespoon chilli flakes, 1 tablespoon olive oil and salt and pepper.
7. Cover and store in the fridge for 4–6 hours.

Quinoa salad

8. Preheat oven to 220 degrees.
9. Cover an ovenproof tray with baking paper and sit to the side.
10. Cut pumpkin into bite size chunks and place in a bowl. Slice red onion into wedges and add to the same bowl.
11. Add the ground coriander, fennel seeds, ground cumin, 1 tablespoon olive oil and salt and pepper to the bowl and mix until evenly coated.
12. Spread the ingredients evenly on the ovenproof tray and roast for approximately 25 minutes.
13. While the pumpkin is cooking, wash the quinoa and add to a small saucepan with ¾ cup of water over medium heat. Cover with a lid and bring to the boil. Once boiling, turn the heat down to low and cook for a further 10 minutes or until the quinoa has absorbed all of the liquid.
14. Once the quinoa is cooked, fluff with a fork, season with salt and pepper and sit to the side the cool.
15. Finely chop the mint and coriander and add to the quinoa along with the 1 tablespoon olive oil, juice of 1 lemon, sumac and salt and pepper. Add the cooked pumpkin and toss gently.
16. Add to a serving plate and garnish with hazelnuts and pepitas.

Prawns

17. Add olive oil to a pan over high heat.
18. Cook prawns for 2 minutes on each side. Remove from the pan and sit to the side.

Assembly

19. Using a serving spoon, serve a single serving of the quinoa salad onto each plate. Position 6–8 prawns on each plate.
20. Eat and enjoy!

Crispy Skin Salmon with Mint Pea Puree and Zucchini Ribbons

|Serves 4|

2 garlic cloves, crushed
2 cups of peas
12 mint leaves
Olive oil
Juice of ½ lemon
2 × salmon fillets, skin on
4 × zucchini, sliced into ribbons
Salt and pepper

Method

Crispy skin salmon

1. Preheat oven to 180 degrees.
2. Cover an ovenproof tray with baking paper and sit to the side.
3. Season salmon fillets with salt and pepper.
4. In a pan over medium heat add olive oil. Place salmon skin side down into the pan and cook until skin is crispy. Rotate to sear remaining sides of the salmon and remove from the heat.
5. Transfer salmon skin side up onto an ovenproof tray and cook in the oven for 12 minutes.
6. While the salmon is cooking, commence making the mint pea puree and zucchini ribbons.

Mint pea puree

7. Heat olive oil in a pan over medium heat. Add 1 clove of garlic (crushed) and peas to the pan and cook for approximately 2–3 minutes or until peas are cooked through.
8. Remove from the heat and add to a food processor with mint leaves, juice of ½ a lemon and salt and pepper.
9. Blend until smooth.
10. Sit to the side with the lid on to retain the heat.
11. Commence cooking the zucchini ribbons.

Zucchini ribbons

12. Heat olive oil in a pan over medium heat. Add garlic, salt and pepper and zucchini ribbons. Sautee until zucchini is cooked. You want the zucchini to still have a slight crunch and hold its form.
13. Remove from the heat.

Assembly

14. Remove the salmon from the oven and sit to the side.
15. Assemble zucchini ribbons and pea puree on the plate.
16. Position salmon skin side up on the plate.
17. Eat and enjoy!

Eye Fillet Steak with Charred Greens, Sweet Potato Mash and Mushroom Sauce

|Serves 4|

4 × 250–300g eye fillet steaks
2 large sweet potatoes, peeled and diced
½ cup pine nuts
1 bunch of broccolini
1 bunch of asparagus
6 large Portobello mushrooms, diced
1 tablespoon butter (or alternative)
½ brown onion, diced
1 clove garlic crushed
¼ cup water
Olive oil
Salt and pepper

Method

Eye fillet

1. Preheat the oven to 180 degrees.
2. Line an ovenproof tray with baking paper and sit to the side.
3. Season the eye fillet with salt and pepper.
4. Add olive oil to a pan over high heat. Add eye fillet to the pan and sear on each side. Be mindful of your pan size that you do not over crowd the pan. You may sear one at a time or if a medium size pan, 2 at a time.
5. Once seared, remove from the heat and place on the ovenproof tray.
6. Cook in the oven for 15 minutes.
7. While the steak is cooking, prepare the vegetables and mushroom puree. If the steak finishes while preparing the vegetables, remove from the heat and rest for 5–10 minutes.

Sweet potato mash

8. Add diced sweet potato to a medium sized saucepan and cover with water. Cook over high heat until sweet potato is soft. Remove from the heat, drain, and season with salt and pepper.
9. Using a hand blender, pulse until the sweet potato is smooth. Sit to the side, covered to retain heat.

Mushroom puree

10. Add ½ brown onion, Portobello mushrooms, butter, and garlic to a pan over medium heat. Cook until the mushrooms soften, and the onion becomes translucent. Add water and cook for a further 2 minutes.
11. Remove from the heat and add to a food processor. Blend until smooth. Cover to retain heat.

Charred greens

12. Add olive oil to a pan over medium to high heat. Add greens and garlic and cook until vegetables are almost cooked through. Add pine nuts and cook for a further minute. The asparagus and broccolini should still have a crunch to it.
13. Remove from the heat.

Assembly

14. Spoon sweet potato mash on the plate. Top with charred green and the mushroom puree. Slice your eye fillet (optional) and position on top of the puree.
15. Eat and enjoy!

Peanut Butter Soup

|Serves 4|

2 packs of Macro chicken nibbles
1 large brown onion, diced
5 large tomatoes, cut into small wedges
5 birds eye chilli, sliced thinly (be mindful of any guests)
1 tablespoon garlic salt
2 tablespoons all purpose seasoning – spicy
Water
1 cup peanut butter

Method

1. In a large saucepan, combine chicken nibbles, onion, tomatoes, chilli, garlic salt and all purpose seasoning. Mix until ingredients are coated evenly.
2. Add enough water to just cover the chicken. Over high heat, cover the saucepan and bring to the boil. Reduce heat to a simmer and cook until the tomatoes are completely soft.
3. Mash the tomatoes until they are blended into the liquid.
4. Add peanut butter and stir until combined. Cook for a further 5–10 minutes until the chicken begins to soften on the bone.
5. Remove from the heat and serve with basmati rice.
6. Enjoy!

Coconut Macadamia Crusted Salmon

|Serves 4|

4 salmon fillets, skinned
¼ cup ground coconut (unsweetened)
¼ cup macadamia nuts, ground
3 tablespoons panko breadcrumbs
Small handful dill, chopped finely
Salt and pepper
1 tablespoon coconut oil
Lemon

Method

1. Preheat oven to 180 degrees. Line a baking tray with baking paper and sit to the side.
2. Season the salmon fillets with salt and pepper and bake in the oven for 5 minutes.
3. While the salmon is baking, add ground coconut, macadamia, breadcrumbs, and dill to a bowl and stir to combine. Add melted coconut oil and stir to combine.
4. Remove the salmon from the oven after 5 minutes and brush lightly with coconut oil. Press the coconut macadamia mixture onto the tops of the fillets.
5. Return salmon to the oven and cook for a further 7 minutes, or until salmon is cooked to your liking.
6. Serve salmon with your choice of salad. This would pair beautifully with a mango and avocado salad.

Lemon Herb Chicken with Roast Vegetable Salad and Smashed Avocado

|Serves 4|

4 chicken breasts, cut into halves to form 8 chicken breast steaks
1 tablespoon fresh garlic, minced
Juice of 4 lemons
2 tablespoons mixed dry herbs
1 red onion
1 tablespoon chilli flakes
2 tablespoons olive oil
Baby spinach
3 avocados, mashed
Pine nuts and pepitas
Salt and pepper
Your choice of vegetables, cut into bite size pieces
(We often will have this meal at the end of the week and use all of our left-over vegetables so we have no waste)

Method

1. In a large bowl, place the chicken, garlic, and juice of 3 lemons, mixed dry herbs, 1 tablespoon olive oil and chilli. Combine until chicken is coated evenly. Cover and store in the fridge overnight.
2. Preheat your oven to 180 degrees. Cover a baking tray with baking paper and sit to the side. Remove chicken from the fridge and sit to the side.
3. In a large bowl, add your vegetables and red onion, salt and pepper and 1 tablespoon olive oil. Stir until the vegetables are coated evenly. Place vegetables on the baking tray and cook in the oven until all vegetables are cooked through. This is usually approximately 25 minutes dependent on the vegetables you choose. Remove from the heat and sit to the side to cool.
4. Line your baking tray again with baking paper and position the chicken evenly. You may need to use two baking trays. Cook the chicken in the oven for 10 minutes.
5. While the chicken is cooking you can start to assemble your salad and mash your avocado. In a bowl add the mashed avocado, remaining lemon juice and salt and pepper to taste. Sit to the side.

6. To assemble your salad, firstly place a small handful of baby spinach on each plate. Sprinkle some pine nuts and pepitas for extra crunch. Top with a large spoonful of the roast vegetables. Repeat this process again.
7. Remove the chicken from the oven once cooked. Position the chicken on top of the salad with a dollop of smashed avocado.
8. Eat and enjoy!

Chilli Prawn and Mango Zoodle Salad

|Serves 4|

1kg uncooked prawns, shells removed
6 zucchinis, made into zoodles
3 ripe mangos, diced
1 tablespoon chilli flakes
1 tablespoon garlic
Juice of 2 lemons
1 tablespoon olive oil
Salt and pepper

Method

1. In a large bowl combine prawns, garlic, chilli, lemon juice, olive oil and salt and pepper. Mix until combined. Cover and store in the fridge for a minimum of 6 hours.
2. In a large pan over medium heat, add olive oil. Cook prawns for 2 minutes per side (medium sized prawns) being careful not to overload the pan. Once all of the prawns are cooked, sit them to the side.
3. Add zoodles to the pan with the remaining juices from the prawns. Toss for 30 seconds while adding in the prawns and diced mango. Remove from the heat.
4. This dish can be served hot or cold. If you prefer to eat the salad cold, store in the fridge for later.
5. Eat and enjoy!

Turkey Lettuce Cups

|Serves 4|

500g Ingham turkey mince
1 capsicum, diced
2 carrots, diced
1 brown onion, chopped finely
⅓ cup honey
⅓ cup organic soy
1 tablespoon chilli flakes
Iceberg lettuce

Method

1. In a pan or wok over medium heat brown turkey mince.
2. Add capsicum, carrots, onion, and chilli and cook until softened.
3. Add soy and honey and cook for a further 5 minutes.
4. Remove from the heat and sit to the side.
5. Separate lettuce leaves and sit to the side.
6. Add a heaped spoonful of the turkey mixture to each lettuce cup.
7. Optional – You may like to serve this with spoonful of basmati rice in each lettuce cup.
8. Eat and enjoy!

Savoury Turkey Mince

|Serves 4|

1 broccoli, chopped finely
1 brown onion, chopped finely
1 capsicum, chopped finely
1 cup peas
2 carrots, chopped finely
8 tomatoes, diced
½ cauliflower, chopped finely
3 tablespoons all purpose seasoning – spicy
5 red chilli, chopped finely
3 tablespoons garlic salt
1-inch ginger, chopped finely
1 cup fresh corn
1 tablespoon olive oil
500g turkey mince

Method

1. In a wok over high heat, add olive oil, onion, chilli, ginger and vegetables.
2. Cook until vegetables begin to soften. Add turkey mince, seasoning and garlic salt and stir to combine.
3. Cook for a further 30 minutes until turkey mince is cooked through and the juices of the vegetables coat the turkey mince.
4. Remove from the heat and serve with basmati rice.
5. Eat and enjoy!

Eggplant Stew

|Serves 4|

3 medium size eggplants, finely diced
500g diced beef
1 brown onion, chopped finely
5 red chilli, chopped finely
3 tablespoons all purpose seasoning – spicy
Olive oil

Method

1. In an airtight container, marinate beef by combining meat with onion, chilli, all purpose seasoning and stir until meat is completely coated then cover for about an hour or two.
2. In a wok over high heat, pour olive oil (just enough to satay the beef) and bring to heat then add meat. Cook until beef is satayed, and all ingredients absorbed then remove and store in an airtight container.
3. In the same wok still over high heat, pour in more olive oil, about a cup. Bring to heat then add in eggplant. Cook eggplant until mushed. Use a masher if necessary, then add in all ingredients from airtight container.
4. Cook for a further 15–20 minutes until all ingredients are absorbed.
5. Remove from heat and serve with basmati rice.
6. Eat and enjoy!

Green Nut Smoothie

1 banana, frozen
1 tablespoon peanut butter
Small handful of baby spinach
½ cup of milk (or alternative, water)
1 teaspoon cinnamon

Method

Add all ingredients to the blender and blend until combined. Pour into your favourite smoothie glass and enjoy!

Berry Delicious Smoothie

1 banana, frozen
½ cup mixed berries
Small handful of baby spinach
1 cup of milk (or alternative, water)

Method

Add all ingredients to the blender and blend until combined. Pour into your favourite smoothie glass and enjoy!

Summer Smoothie

1 banana, frozen
1 mango cheek
¼ cup blueberries
Small handful of baby spinach
1 cup of milk (or alternative, water)

Method

Add all ingredients to the blender and blend until combined. Pour into your favourite smoothie glass and enjoy!

Choco-nut Smoothie

1 banana, frozen
2 medjool dates
½ tablespoon cacao
1 tablespoon peanut butter
½ cup milk (or alternative, water)

Method

Add all ingredients to the blender and blend until combined. Pour into your favourite smoothie glass and enjoy!

Mixed Berry Bliss Balls

1 cup fresh strawberries and blueberries
10 medjool dates, tones removed
1 cup raw cashews
1 cup desiccated coconut
Pinch of salt

Method

1. Place all of the ingredients into your food processor and pulse at high speed until the mixture is broken down, well combined and sticking together. Use your hands to shape the mixture into balls.
2. Roll the balls in coconut (optional) and place in the fridge to set.
3. Eat and enjoy!

Crunchy Nut Bliss Balls

¼ cup coconut
¼ cup raw cashews
10 medjool dates, tones removed
½ cup crunchy peanut butter
¼ cup cacao
1 tablespoon honey (optional)
¼ cup crushed peanuts
Pinch of salt

Method

1. Place all the ingredients into your food processor and blend until the mixture is combined and sticking together. Use your hands to press and shape the mixture into balls and place the balls into the fridge to set.
2. Eat and enjoy!

Choc Peppermint Bliss Balls

1 cup dry roasted almonds
1 cup dry roasted cashews
10 medjool dates
3 tablespoons cacao
12 fresh mint leaves
Pinch of salt
Water

Method

1. Place all the ingredients into your food processor and pulse at high speed until the mixture is broken down, well combined and sticking together. If the mixture is too dry, add a small amount of water and pulse until the ingredients are sticking together.
2. Use your hands to shape the mixture into balls. Store in the fridge in an airtight container or in the freezer.
3. Eat and enjoy!

Lemon Bliss Balls

1 cup dry roasted cashews
1 cup coconut flakes
5 medjool dates
1 tablespoon honey
Juice of 2 lemons
Pinch of salt
Water

Method

1. Place all the ingredients into your food processor and pulse at high speed until the mixture is broken down, well combined and sticking together. If the mixture is too dry, add a small amount of water and pulse until the ingredients are sticking together.
2. Use your hands to shape the mixture into balls. Store in the fridge in an airtight container or in the freezer.
3. Eat and enjoy!

Mint Pea Puree

1 garlic clove, crushed
2 cups peas
8–12 mint leaves
Juice of ½ lemon
Salt and pepper
Olive oil

Method

1. Heat olive oil in a pan over medium heat. Add garlic and peas to the pan and cook for approximately 2–3 minutes or until peas are cooked through.
2. Remove from the heat and add to a food processer with mint leaves, lemon juice and salt and pepper.
3. Blend until smooth.
4. Serve with your choice of protein and vegetables.

Mushroom Sauce

1 garlic clove, crushed
1 tablespoon butter
6 Portobello mushrooms, sliced
Salt and pepper
Water
½ brown onion, chopped finely

Method

1. Add onion, Portobello mushrooms, butter, and garlic to a pan over medium heat. Cook until the mushrooms soften, and the onion becomes translucent. Add water and cook for a further 2 minutes.
2. Remove from the heat and add to a food processor. Blend until smooth.
3. Season with salt and pepper to taste.
4. Serve with your choice of protein and vegetables.

APPENDIX B
CORRECT TECHNIQUES AND FORMS FOR SOME COMMON EXERCISES

Here are some correct techniques and forms for some common exercises.

RUNNING

Running is not just getting up, putting on a pair of shoes, getting out the door and putting one foot in front of the other. Though it seems that simple, there are some things to consider to help you avoid injuries. Due to its repetitive nature, injuries are quite common with running, and even seasoned runners and coaches do experience this from time to time. Here are some steps to help you minimise your risk of getting injured:

- **Look ahead of you.** Do not watch your feet. Aim to look about three to six metres ahead of you. It helps you keep your head up and see what is coming.

- **Make sure your posture is upright and straight.** Keep your head up, shoulders relaxed, and back straight. Do not lean forward or backward; this can cause fatigue. Continue to check your posture. As you fatigue towards the end of your run, your form can start to go out the window, which can lead to neck, shoulder, and lower back pain.

- **Do not round your shoulders.** Keep them square and facing forward. Rounding your shoulders can tighten the chest and restrict breathing.

- **Swing your arms from your shoulders not from your elbows.** Drive your elbows back and let them swing forward.

- **Keep your hands beside your waist.** Keep your hands at waist level where they might lightly graze your hips with every stride. Hold your arms at about 90-degree angle. Holding them any higher may cause fatigue and tightness in shoulders.

- **Do not swing your arms across your chest.** Keep them by your side. Swinging your arms across your chest can cause you to rotate through the hips and slouch, which can lead to inefficient breathing, which can also cause stiches and cramps.

- **Do not toe or heel strike.** Land midfoot. Landing toes first will fatigue your calves and landing heels first does not only mean overstriding but will also put the brakes on and can lead to wasted energy and can sometimes cause injury.

- **Try not to bounce.** Keep your stride close to the ground and take short, light steps as though you were stepping on a hotbed of coals. Bouncing up and down wastes too much energy and can be hard on the body.

- **Do not clench your fists.** Relax your hands and arms as much as possible. Clenching your fists can cause tightness in your arms as well as waste energy.

- **Get fitted with the right running shoes that suit the shape of your feet.** Having the wrong shoes can lead to injuries. Also, depending on how often you run, change shoes frequently. Your running shoes should not be your everyday shoes. If unsure, see a podiatrist.

BENCH PRESS

Bench press is an upper-body strength training exercise that works – for the sake of simplicity – the muscles of your chest as well as other supporting muscles like your shoulders and arms. Having correct technique when performing the bench press is crucial to success, and it also helps to prevent injuries which can sometimes be severe.

Lie in a supine position (face up) on a flat bench and grab weight (generally a barbell although dumbbells can be used too) in both hands; lower weight to chest level and press up until arms are extended back to starting position – that is one repetition, or rep as it is known for short.

SQUATS

Squats are one of my favourite exercises to do. Even though the squat is regarded as a lower body exercise, it is a compound exercise that works your whole body, with the focus being primarily on the muscles of the thighs, buttocks, and hamstrings. It also helps to strengthen the bones, ligaments, and tendons of the lower body. It is a compound exercise because it moves through various joints, including the hip, knee, and ankle joints. The squat, when performed with the correct form or technique, works your core muscles, lower back, abdominals, upper back, shoulders, arms and more.

There are various types of squats – here are some examples and how to perform them correctly:

- **Body weight squat:** performed without weights. Stand with feet slightly wider than shoulder-width apart with toes slightly pointing out; keep your knees in line with your toes; keep your back flat and head in a neutral position; with arms straight out or crossed in front of your chest, hinge at the hips and bend at the knee and ankle joints until your hips are just below your knees and then stand back up to starting position.

- **Back squat:** same form as the body weight squat except this time with a barbell across your back and you use your hands to hold onto the barbell. The bar can be placed in two positions: high bar – upper across your trapezius muscle just below your neck; or low bar – lower across your upper back near your rear deltoids. It's called a back squat – not a neck squat. Do not place the bar on your neck as I see many people do.

- **Front squat:** hold a barbell in front of your body across your clavicles or deltoids, either in a clean grip or with arms crossed with hands placed on top of the bar, and squat down and stand upright.

- **Sumo squat:** can be performed with barbell, dumbbell, or kettlebell; stand with feet wider than shoulder width apart with toes and knees pointing outward, squat down, and stand upright.

- **Goblet squat:** performed with either a kettlebell or dumbbell held with both hands in front of you across your chest.

- **Box squat:** at the bottom of your squat, you sit on a box or bench.

- **Hack squat:** performed with heels joined together and a barbell held in the hands just behind the legs.

- **Overhead squat:** is performed with the barbell held overhead in a wide-arm snatch grip.

- **Split squat:** can be referred to as a static lunge. Take one step forward and drop the knee of the rear leg as close to the ground as possible and stand back up. This can also be performed with the rear leg raised up onto a platform about knee high: the exercise is then called Bulgarian split squat.

- **Jump squat:** performed by squatting down and at the bottom of the squat jumping up.

- **Zercher squat:** performed by holding the barbell in the bend of your elbows.

- **Pistol squat:** a body weight squat performed with one leg to full depth with the other leg extended in front of you off the ground.

- **Smith squat:** a squat performed using the Smith machine.

DEADLIFTS

If I had to pick one exercise as my favourite exercise out of them all, it would have to be the deadlift, and that is simply because of the number of muscles you work when you do deadlifts. Though seen as a lower-body exercise, it is very much a full-body exercise. At any given time, there are at least 30 different muscles in your body that are put to work when you do the deadlift correctly. From the muscles in your feet to the ones in your hands, lower back, hamstrings, glutes (butt muscles), thigh muscles, abdominals, shoulders, neck, arms – they all work to help you complete the movement.

As the name suggests, a deadlift is performed by lifting a loaded barbell off the ground. The weight must be dead; that is, without any momentum. There are three phases to doing a deadlift: the setup, drive, and lockout. Like the squat, there are also different variations of the deadlifts:

- **Traditional deadlift:**
  - *The setup:* stand behind a loaded bar with feet at about hip-width apart; stand close to the bar so it is just touching or nearly touching your legs; keep your feet flat on the ground; hinge or bend at the hips keeping your weight in your heels; maintain a flat back as you hinge your hips back; make sure your knees are in line with your toes and not tracking forward over them; grip the bar outside of your legs and pull your shoulders back to engage your lats to generate more force from your erectors.

  - *The drive:* keep your back muscles contracted to maintain a safe posture throughout the movement; pretend as though you were standing on a coin lying flat and your goal is to push it into the ground with your heels; drive up and forward with your hips and legs to stand up straight as you lift the weight off the floor; take a deep breath and hold it while you lift the weight to stabilise your core.

  - *The lockout:* finish the movement by driving your hips into the bar and stand upright and as tall as possible; contract your glutes and abdominal muscles to protect your lower back. Breath out at the top of your motion.

To lower the bar, perform all the steps above in reverse. Keep your back and core muscles tight, hinge at the hips and knees, and keep the bar close; lower your chest down to your knees to bring the bar down.

- **Sumo deadlift:** the difference between the traditional deadlift and the Sumo deadlift is that you grip the bar inside of your legs instead of outside and you take a wide stance – wider than shoulder-width apart with your toes pointing out at about 45 degrees.

- **Romanian deadlift:** nowadays commonly referred to as RDL by hipsters, this is a variation of the traditional deadlift but unlike it, the Romanian deadlift is performed with a slight bend in your knees – as you hinge your hips back, you lower the bar to just below your knees, maintaining a straight spine, and then stand back up to starting position.

- **Stiff-legged deadlift:** much like the Romanian deadlift but the major difference lies within the range of motion. With the stiff-legged deadlift, you can go lower to the ground or just off the ground whereas with the Romanian deadlift you hinge down until the bar is just below your knees and then you stand back up.

APPENDIX C
EXERCISE PROGRAMS

At home, anywhere and anytime – these are body weight exercises designed to help you get the desired results of exercise with zero equipment.

Beginner

1. Body weight squats

2. Push-ups

3. Sit-ups

4. Star jumps

Program 1A – perform each exercise individually for 10–12 repetitions by 3–5 sets then move on to the next exercise and repeat until you have done them all.

Program 1B – perform each exercise for 10–12 repetitions back to back without any break until you have done them all. Have 1–2 minutes break then repeat for 3–5 sets.

Program 2A – perform each exercise for 30 seconds and do as many repetitions as you can within that time. Have 15 seconds break then move on to the next exercise until you have done them all. Have 1– 2 minutes break then repeat for 3–5 sets.

Program 2B – perform each exercise for 30 seconds and do as many repetitions as you can within that time, without any break. Move on to the next exercise until you have done them all. Have 1–2 minutes break then repeat for 3–5 sets.

Program 3 – perform each exercise for 20 seconds and do as many repetitions as you can within that time. Have 10 seconds break and repeat 8 times before moving on to the next exercise. Have about 1–2 minutes break in between exercises.

Intermediate to advanced

M 13 × burpees

U 21 × jump squats

S 19 × push-ups

C 3 × 15m frog jumps

L 12 per side mountain climbers

E 5 × 15m sprints

G 7 per side jump lunges

A 1 minute plank

R 18 × star jumps

D 4 × 15m bear crawls

E 5 per side plank push-ups

N 14 per side cross crunches

Program 1 – perform each exercise for the number of reps back to back with minimum to no break. After MUSCLE, have 1–2 minutes break then perform GARDEN. Repeat for 2–5 sets.

Program 2 – perform each exercise for time – 45 seconds ON and 15 seconds OFF. Do as many repetitions as you can within 45 seconds. Have 15 seconds break and then move on to the next exercise. After completing MUSCLE, have 1–2 minutes break before doing GARDEN. Complete MUSCLE GARDEN for at least 2 sets or 3–5 sets depending on your level of fitness.

Animal movement – bear crawls, inch worm, inch worm with push-ups, ape walk, duck walk, crab walk, cheetah sprint, crocodile walk.

Kettle-bell workout (two-handed) – this workout can also be done at home. You may need to buy a kettlebell from your local sporting store.

1. Kettlebell upright row
2. Kettlebell overhead press
3. Kettlebell deadlifts
4. Kettlebell swings
5. Kettlebell squat and press
6. Kettlebell deadlift into upright row
7. Kettlebell russian twist

Program 1A – perform each exercise individually for 10–12 repetitions for 3–5 sets then move on to the next exercise and repeat until you have done them all.

Program 1B – perform each exercise for 10–12 repetitions back to back without any break until you have done them all. Have 1–2 minutes break then repeat for 3–5 sets.

Program 2A – perform each exercise for 30 seconds and do as many repetitions as you can within that time, have 15 seconds break then move on to the next exercise until you have done them all. Have 1–2 minutes break then repeat for 3–5 sets.

Below are some training programs that you can do in the gym.

PROGRAM 1

Workout 1
Upper Body – Weights

Warmup – 5–10 minutes on rowing machine

Chest
Chest press – 12–15 reps × 3 sets
Incline press – 12–15 reps × 3 sets

Back
Lat pulldowns – 12–15 reps × 3 sets
Seated row – 12–15 reps × 3 sets

Shoulders
Shoulder press – 12–15 reps × 3 sets
Kettlebell upright rows – 12–15 reps × 3 sets

Biceps
Barbell biceps curls – 12–15 reps × 3 sets
Dumbbell bicep curls – 12–15 reps × 3 sets

Triceps
Cable tricep push-downs – 12–15 reps × 3 sets
Dumbbell tricep extensions – 12–15 reps × 3 sets

Cooldown – stretch

Workout 2

Lower Body – Weights

Warmup – 5–10 minutes on bike

Legs
Leg press – 12–15 reps × 3 sets
Leg extensions – 12–15 reps × 3 sets
Leg curls – 12–15 reps × 3 sets
Hip adduction – 12–15 reps × 3 sets

Glutes
Weighted bridges – 12–15 reps × 3 sets
Hip abduction – 12–15 reps × 3 sets

Lower back
Romanian deadlifts – 12–15 reps × 3 sets
Back extensions – 12–15 reps × 3 sets

Calves
Seated calf raises – 12–15 reps × 3 sets
Standing calf raises – 12–15 reps × 3 sets

Cooldown – stretch

Workout 3

Cardio
45 minutes of cardio – walk, jog, run, row, ride, cross trainer,
stair climb

Workout 4

Functional Fitness – Circuit

Warmup – 5–10 minutes on cross trainer

1. One arm kettlebell squat – 10 reps per side
2. One arm dumbbell lunge and press – 10 reps per side
3. One arm kettlebell swing – 10 reps per side
4. One arm dumbbell clean and press – 10 reps per side
5. Walking lunges with wall ball, lunge, twist, and bounce – 10 reps per side
6. Russian twists with wall ball or medicine ball – 10 reps per side × 3–5 sets

Workout 5

Core

Warmup – 5–10 minute run

1. Mountain climbers – 3 × 30 sec rounds
2. Sit-ups/crunches – 3 × 15 reps
3. Bicycle crunches – 3 × 20 reps – 10 per side
4. Toe taps – 3 × 20 reps
5. Prone planks – 3 × 45 seconds
6. Side planks – 3 × 30 seconds
7. Butt-ups – 3 × 10 reps
8. Cross crunches – 3 × 20 reps – 10 per side
9. Leg raises – 3 × 10 reps
10. Russian twists – 10 per side

PROGRAM 2

Workout 1

Upper Body – Weights

Warmup – 10 minutes on rowing machine

Chest
Barbell bench press – 10–12 reps × 3 sets
Dumbbell incline press – 10–12 reps × 3 sets

Back
Assisted chin-ups – 10–12 reps × 3 sets
Single arm d'bell row – 10–12 reps × 3 sets

Shoulders
Barbell military press – 10–12 reps × 3 sets
D'bell upright rows – 10–12 reps × 3 sets

Biceps
Cable biceps curls – 10–12 reps × 4 sets
D'bell hammer curls – 10–12 reps × 3 sets

Triceps
Triceps dips – 10–12 reps × 4 sets
D'bell triceps kickbacks – 10–12 reps × 3 sets

Cooldown – stretch

Workout 2

Lower Body – Weights

Warmup – 10 minutes upright bike/stairs

Legs
Back/goblet squats – 10–12 reps × 3 sets
D'bell walking lunges – 10–12 reps × 3 sets
Hip thrusters – 10–12 reps × 3 sets
D'bell side lunges – 10–12 reps × 3 sets
D'bell jump squats – 10–12 reps × 3 sets
D'bell jump lunges – 10–12 reps × 3 sets

Lower back
Stiff-legged deadlifts – 10–12 reps × 3 sets
Good mornings – 10–12 reps × 3 sets

Calves
Seated calf raises – 10–12 reps × 4 sets
Standing calf raises – 10–12 reps × 4 sets

Cooldown – stretch

Workout 3

Cardio

Warmup – 2 min row

Sprints – 30 seconds ON 30 seconds OFF

1. Rowing machine

2. Air-bike

3. Cross trainer

4. Battle ropes

× 5–10 rounds on each machine

Workout 4

Functional Fitness – Circuit

Warmup – 10 minutes on air-bike/cross trainer

1. Burpees
2. Dumbbell thrusters/squat press
3. Kettle-bell swings
4. B'bell deadlift into upright rows
5. Ball slams
6. Push-ups
7. 1 Minute sprint on rower

12 reps × 2 or more sets

Workout 5

Core

Warmup – 10 minutes total of high knees, skipping and star jumps

1. Knee crunch – 3 × 10 reps
2. Pulse-ups – 3 × 10 reps
3. Star plank – 3 × 45 seconds
4. Heel taps – 3 × 10 reps per side
5. Plank crunches – 3 × 10 reps per side
6. Climber taps – 3 × 10 reps per side

Cooldown – stretch

PROGRAM 3

Workout 1

Chest and Triceps – Weights

Warmup – 5 minutes on air-bike

Chest

D'bell chest press – 8–10 reps × 4 sets
Barbell incline press – 8–10 reps × 4 sets
Machine chest press – 8–10 reps × 4 sets
Machine incline press – 8–10 reps × 4 sets
D'bell chest flys – 8–10 reps × 4 sets (flat bench)

Triceps

Triceps dips – 8–10 reps × 4 sets
D'bell triceps kickbacks – 8–10 reps × 4 sets
Cable triceps push-downs – 8–10 reps × 4 sets
D'bell triceps extensions – 8–10 reps × 4 sets

Cooldown – 50 sit-ups

Workout 2

Back and Biceps – Weights

Warmup – 5 minutes on rowing machine

Back

Assisted chin-ups – 8–10 reps × 4 sets
Single arm d'bell row – 8–10 reps × 4 sets
Machine lat pulldown – 8–10 reps × 4 sets
Seated row – 8–10 reps × 4 sets
Seated d'bell back flys – 8–10 reps × 4 sets (45 degrees incline
bench – facing down)

Biceps

Barbell biceps curls – 8–10 reps × 4 sets
Dumbbell bicep curls – 8–10 reps × 4 sets
Cable biceps curls – 8–10 reps × 4 sets
D'bell hammer curls – 8–10 reps × 4 sets

Cooldown – 50 per side bicycle crunches

Workout 3

Legs and Shoulders – Weights

Warmup – 5 minutes air-bike

Legs

Barbell back squats – 8–10 reps × 4 sets
D'bell deadlifts – 8–10 reps × 4 sets
Leg press – 8–10 reps × 4 sets
D'bell walking lunges – 8–10 reps (per side) × 4 sets
Seated calf raises – Failure × 4 sets

Shoulders

D'bell shoulder press – 8–10 reps × 4 sets
Barbell upright rows – 8–10 reps × 4 sets
Machine shoulder press – 8–10 reps × 4 sets
D'bell lateral raises – 8–10 reps × 4 sets

Cooldown – Mountain climbers – 4 × 30 seconds

Workout 4

Cardio

30–60 minutes jog (slow but sure. If you have got bad knees, ride)

Workout 5

Functional Fitness – Circuit

Warmup – 5–10 minutes on cross trainer

M 13 × burpees

U 21 × jump squats

S 19 × push-ups

C 3 × 15m frog jumps

L 12 kettlebell swings

E 5 × 15m sled push

G 7 per side jump lunges

A 1 minute plank

R 18 × dead ball slams

D 4 × 15m bear crawls

E 5 per side plank push-ups

N 14 sit-outs/kick-throughs

× 2–3 full sets of MUSCLE and GARDEN

PROGRAM 4

Workout 1

Full Body – Weights and Body Weight Combo

Warmup – 5 minutes on rowing machine

Bench/chest press vs burpees – 2 super sets at 12 reps, 10 reps and 8 reps

Chin-ups/lat pulldowns vs kettlebell swings – 2 super sets at 12 reps, 10 reps and 8 reps

Cable biceps curls vs triceps pushdowns – 2 super sets at 12 reps, 10 reps and 8 reps

Workout 2

Full Body – Weights and Body Weight Combo

Warmup – 5 minutes on air-bike

Squat/leg press vs overhead ball slams – 2 super sets at 12 reps, 10 reps and 8 reps

Barbell push presses vs box jumps – 2 super sets at 12 reps, 10 reps and 8 reps

Barbell deadlifts vs tyre flips – 2 super sets at 12 reps, 10 reps and 8 reps

Workout 3

REST or Active Recovery

Walk, jog, row, cross train or ride at a moderate intensity for 30–45 minutes

Workout 4

Core

Warmup – 10 min run

1. Mountain climbers – 3 × 30 sec rounds
2. Sit-ups or crunches – 3 × 15 reps
3. Bicycle crunches – 3 × 20 reps – 10 per side
4. Toe taps – 3 × 20 reps
5. Prone planks – 3 × 45 seconds
6. Side planks – 3 × 30 seconds
7. Butt-ups – 3 × 10 reps
8. Cross crunches – 3 × 20 reps – 10 per side
9. Leg raises – 3 × 10 reps
10. Russian twists – 10 per side × 3 sets

Workout 5

Full Body – Legs and Shoulders Combo

Warmup – 10 minutes on cross trainer

1. Barbell thrusters – 10 reps × 5 sets
2. Barbell deadlift into upright row – 10 reps × 5 sets
3. Barbell clean and press – 10 reps × 5 sets
4. Lunges into lateral raises – 10 reps × 5 sets
5. Bus driver – 30 seconds × 5 sets

These exercise programs have been carefully designed to take you on a journey. I may not know you, what you can or cannot do; as such, it is your responsibility to figure out what your abilities are and proceed with caution. Do what you can within the time that you can afford, but above all do something.

Note: Where I have mentioned 'machine' I am referring to either a pin-loaded machine (machines where you add or remove weights using a pin) or plate-loaded machines (machines where you add or remove weights using plates).